Hayette Sénia BENSABER
Fedwa ADDOU

Triple-negative breast cancer in young women in western Algeria

Hayette Sénia BENSABER
Fedwa ADDOU

Triple-negative breast cancer in young women in western Algeria

Triple negative unfavorable prognosis

ScienciaScripts

Imprint
Any brand names and product names mentioned in this book are subject to trademark, brand or patent protection and are trademarks or registered trademarks of their respective holders. The use of brand names, product names, common names, trade names, product descriptions etc. even without a particular marking in this work is in no way to be construed to mean that such names may be regarded as unrestricted in respect of trademark and brand protection legislation and could thus be used by anyone.

Cover image: www.ingimage.com

This book is a translation from the original published under ISBN 978-620-6-70450-8.

Publisher:
Sciencia Scripts
is a trademark of
Dodo Books Indian Ocean Ltd. and OmniScriptum S.R.L publishing group

120 High Road, East Finchley, London, N2 9ED, United Kingdom
Str. Armeneasca 28/1, office 1, Chisinau MD-2012, Republic of Moldova, Europe
Managing Directors: Ieva Konstantinova, Victoria Ursu
info@omniscriptum.com

Printed at: see last page
ISBN: 978-620-8-39419-6

Contents

SUMMARY

Triple-negative breast cancer represents a particular group of breast carcinomas defined immunohistochemically by the absence of hormone receptor expression and the absence of HER2 receptor overexpression. This group of tumours, which have the poorest prognosis, does not currently benefit from any targeted treatment, and the only validated systemic therapy is chemotherapy.

This is a retrospective study of the last six years carried out at the Etablissement Hôspitalier Universitaire d'Oran "1er Novembre 1954" (EHUO) between 2017 and 2022 involving 59 young patients with triple-negative invasive breast carcinomas.

Anatomopathologically, infiltrating ductal carcinoma is the most predominant type, representing 86.4% of cases, with a majority T2 tumour size of 66.1%. Histopronostic grades II and III each accounted for 66.1% and 33.9% of cases.

Axillary lymph node metastases occurred in 88.1% of cases. In terms of treatment, 10.2% of patients underwent conservative treatment and 89.8% underwent radical surgery of the Patey type.

Despite advances in treatment and the advent of targeted therapies, breast cancer remains the leading cause of death in women. Current clinical and histological classifications do not allow us to fully establish the prognostic and predictive parameters of response to treatment.

Keywords : Breast cancer ,triple negative ,young woman,poor prognosis,metastasis , progesterone(PR) , (rstrogen(RE), protein (HER2) , mastectomy .

GENERAL INTRODUCTION

In most countries, breast cancer is the most common cancer in women. Every year, more than a million new cases occur worldwide, representing 30% of female cancer cases in industrialised countries and 14% in developing countries. It is also the leading cause of cancer-related death in women, with 410,000 deaths annually **(Rochefort H et *al.*, 2008)**.

It is defined as any primary malignant neoplastic proliferation originating from the mammary parenchyma, and is the most frequently diagnosed cancer in women worldwide, affecting one in 9 women during their lifetime and causing 1 in 27 deaths. It is the leading cancer in women and its incidence is rising steadily; it is seen in women between the ages of 35 and 55, with early forms becoming increasingly common in Algeria. It is exceptional in men (1%) and generally develops on gynaecomastia or klinfelter's syndrome **(Boughera N, 2012)**.

The diversity of clinical presentations, responses to treatment and prognosis of breast cancer can be explained by a high degree of histological and molecular heterogeneity.

In clinical practice, the different subtypes of breast cancer are estimated using immunohistochemical (IHC) tests for hormone receptors (HR) (estrogen and progesterone receptors) and the oncoprotein HER2 (human epidermal growth factor receptor-2); these tests are carried out on all cases of invasive breast cancer.

One type of breast cancer has attracted a great deal of interest over the last fifteen years: Triple-negative breast cancer (TNBC), which is defined by the absence of hormone receptor expression, and the absence of HER2 oncoprotein amplification/overexpression, accounts for 12-17% of breast cancers **(Naibo P, 2018).**

Most triple-negative breast cancers are invasive ductal carcinomas (IDC). Ductal carcinoma in situ (DCIS) can also be triple negative.

Currently, triple-negative breast cancer is diagnosed via a two-stage imaging and immunohistochemistry (IHC) procedure, which is operator-dependent and can be time-consuming. There is therefore a crucial need to develop rapid, advanced technologies to improve diagnostic efficiency.

CSTN triple-negative breast cancers show similarities to cancers developed in the setting of a constitutional deleterious mutation in the BRCA 1 gene, pointing to potential new therapeutic avenues **(Naibo P, 2018).**

Triple-negative breast cancer usually responds well to chemotherapy. However, its risk of recurrence (recurrence) in the five years following treatment is high compared with hormone receptor-positive or HER2-positive breast cancer. This risk decreases after five years.

The objectives of this study are :

- ✓ Describe the clinico-epidemiological and histopronostic features of the disease,
- ✓ To analyse changes in the pathology of triple-negative breast cancer over the last six years.
- ✓ To improve the diagnosis and individual prognosis of patients aged 50 and under suffering from this pathology in the population of western Algeria.

CHAPTER I

PATHOLOGICAL BREAST

I.1 Definition

The breast is made up of a mammary gland, support fibres (Cooper's ligaments) and fat (adipose tissue), all covered by the skin. The quantity of each of these components can vary from one woman to another. The breast is located above the pectoral muscle. The breast also contains nerves and blood and lymph vessels. The mammary gland is divided into 15 to 20 sections called "lobes", made up of lobules. These are connected to ducts that run under the nipple (located in the centre of the breast). Lymph nodes can also be seen, filtering out microbes and protecting the body against infection and disease. Breast cancer can develop in both a milk duct and a lobule, and can also be found in the lymph nodes **[1]**.

The breast can be affected by benign or malignant pathologies. In order to detect them early, it is advisable to carry out regular self-examinations to feel for the presence of any mammary lymph nodes.

Self-examination, also known as autopalpation, involves examining the breasts to detect changes that could point towards a diagnosis of cancer, and should be carried out once a month from the age of 25. Self-examination does not replace a clinical examination by a doctor, and certainly not a mammogram **[2]**.

If a patient has felt anything strange, she should make an appointment to see her GP or gynaecologist. The doctor or gynaecologist will palpate the breasts again. He or she may order further tests, such as a mammogram if the patient is over 30, an ultrasound scan, a breast MRI or a blood test. And don't forget to see a GP or gynaecologist once a year, because breast self-examination is no substitute for a consultation with a health professional **(Figure 1) [2]**.

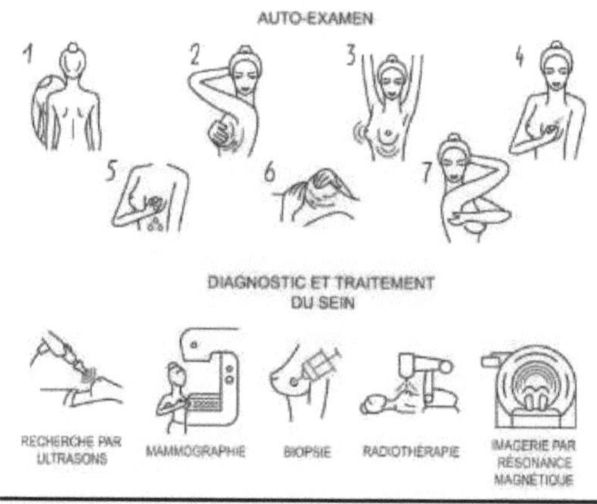

Figure 1: Tests to diagnose breast cancer [2].

1.1.1 Benign breast diseases

1.1.1.1 Breast calcifications

Corresponding to calcium deposits in the breast tissue, which are not correlated with the presence or absence of cancer, the radiologist examines their size, shape and arrangement using mammography. Some of their characteristics, such as an irregular shape or certain groupings, may be suspicious **[3].**

1.1.1.2 Benign conditions

These diseases of the breast are not synonymous with breast cancer, and do not generally involve any vital danger for the patient, such as cysts, nipple discharge, atypical hyperplasia, pain, adenosis, fat necrosis, gynaecomastia (in men), ectasia of the milk ducts, etc **[3].**

1.1.1.3 Non-cancerous tumours

It is a mass that does not spread to other parts of the body (no metastases). It is not usually life-threatening. It is usually surgically removed and does not usually recur, such as fibroadenosis, intracanal papilloma, phyllodes tumour, and non-cancerous tumours such as lipoma, adenoma, neurofibroma, haemangioma, hamartoma, granular cell tumour **[3].**

1.1.2 Malignant breast diseases

1.1.2.1 Ductal carcinoma

The most common forms in the glandular cells of the mammary ducts, and may be in situ (present only in the mammary ducts) or infiltrating (extending into neighbouring mammary tissue) **[4]**.

1.1.2.2 Lobular carcinoma

It originates in the lobules of the breast, then crosses these lobules and invades neighbouring breast tissue. It can also spread (metastasise) to lymph nodes and other parts of the body **[4].**

1.1.2.3 Inflammatory breast cancer

Inflammatory breast cancer is rare (1-5% of all cases) and aggressive, which means that it develops and spreads rapidly. The cancer cells block the lymphatic vessels in the skin of the breast. It is called "inflammatory" because the affected breast appears inflamed (red and swollen). IBC develops and spreads rapidly and is considered locally advanced breast cancer when the cancer cells have invaded nearby tissue or lymph nodes **[5].**

1.1.2.4 Paget's disease

Paget's disease of the breast is a rare type of breast cancer. It appears as a rash or other changes on the skin of the nipple, usually on one breast. Paget's disease of the breast is more common in women over the age of 50 **[6].**

1.1.3 Stages of carcinogenesis

Research in endocrinology led to the first targeted cancer therapies using antiestrogens. Breast cancer cell lines have made it possible to elucidate the mechanisms of the mitogenic effect of estrogens, the basis of their activity as tumour-promoting agents **[7]**. Experiments carried out on cell models show that carcinogenesis can be divided schematically into three phases:

1.1.3.1 Initiation

Is a one-off step corresponding to an alteration in the genome of a normal cell, giving it the property of escaping cellular regulation: DNA alterations of endogenous origin (errors during DNA duplication), the effect of free radicals on DNA, alterations induced by carcinogenic environmental factors. A DNA alteration (mutation) is only transmitted to cells derived from the "initiated" cell if it is not destined to die and if the DNA alterations are not repaired **[8].**

1.1.3.2 Promotion

Is a relatively long phase during which the initiated cell proliferates and gradually leads to the development of mutated cells. Various endogenous factors (growth factors and hormones) or exogenous factors (chemical toxins, dietary factors, etc.), due to their repetitive action, will deregulate some of the mechanisms controlling cell multiplication **[8].**

1.1.3.3 Progress

This is a complex phase consisting of the vascularisation of the tumour (Angiogenesis) and the acquisition of the capacity to invade (Metastasis) **[8].**

1.1.3.3.1 Angiogenesis

Is the formation of new blood vessels from existing ones. To proliferate, cancer cells need a supply of nutrients and oxygen. The tumour will therefore trigger the creation of new blood vessels.

1.1.3.3.2 Metastasis

A tumour formed from cancer cells that have broken away from an initial tumour (primary tumour) and migrated via lymphatic vessels or blood vessels to another part of the body, where they have taken up residence. Metastases tend to develop in the lungs, liver, bones or brain. It is not another cancer, but the original cancer that has spread. For example, a metastasis of breast cancer to the lung is a tumour made up of breast cells; it is not lung cancer. The risk of developing metastases depends on the characteristics of the initial tumour.

CHAPTER II

EPIDEMIOLOGY OF BREAST CANCER

11.1 Descriptive epidemiology

11.1.1. On a global scale

In 2020, they counted 2.3 million women with breast cancer and 685,000 deaths from breast cancer worldwide.

By the end of 2020, 7.8 million women had been diagnosed with breast cancer in the last five years, making breast cancer the most common cancer worldwide.

Worldwide, women lose more years of life (disability-adjusted life expectancy) to breast cancer than to any other type of cancer. Breast cancer occurs in every country in the world and affects women of all ages from puberty onwards (although the incidence rate increases with age) **[9].**

Although incidence is rising in most parts of the world, there are huge inequalities between rich and poor countries **(Figure 2) [10]**.

These trends are largely explained by the fact that low- and middle-income countries have had to focus their limited health resources on combating infectious diseases and improving maternal and child health, while their health services are not equipped to prevent, diagnose and treat cancers. This is due to a lack of early detection and access to treatment **(Figure 3) [10]**.

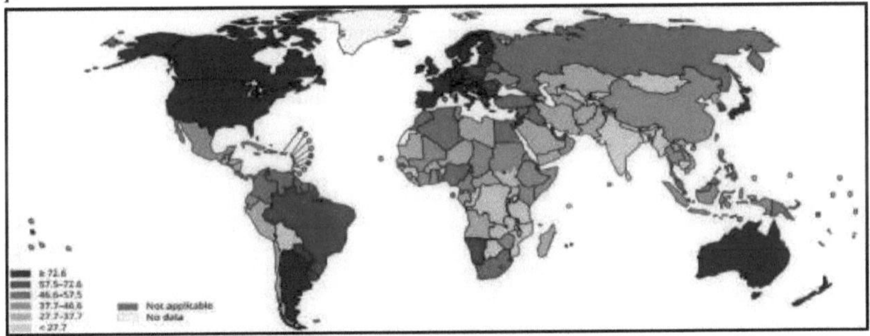

Figure 2: Worldwide age-standardised incidence rates of breast cancer (GLOBOCAN 2020) [10].

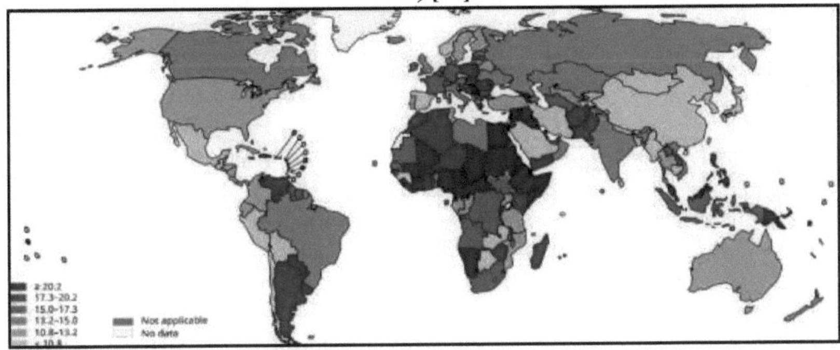

Figure 3: Worldwide age-standardised mortality rates for breast cancer (GLOBOCAN 2020) [10].

11.1.2. On a national scale

Breast cancer is the most common cancer in Algeria, and its incidence continues to rise, with the average age of onset in Algeria being 48. Breast cancer is the leading cause of cancer in Algeria, with 2.26 million new cases per year, followed by lung cancer (2.2 million), colorectal cancer (1.93 million), prostate cancer (1.41 million), skin cancer (1.2 million) and stomach cancer (1.09 million), according to GLOBOCAN 20202 **(Figure 4)[9].**

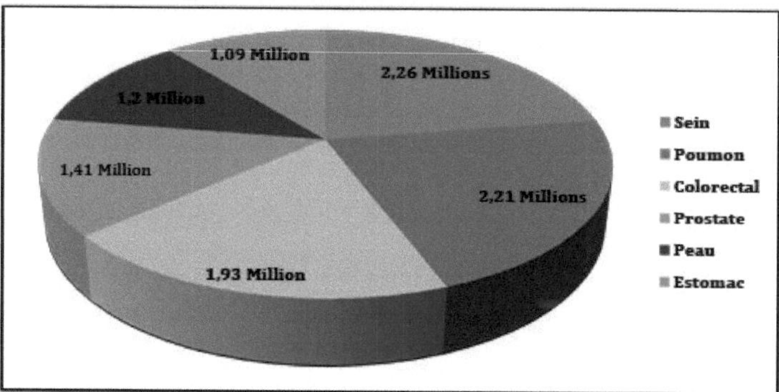

Figure 4: Number of registered cases of breast cancer in Algeria in 2020 [9] Breast cancer is the most frequently diagnosed cancer, followed by colorectal and lung cancer (in terms of incidence) and vice versa (in terms of mortality), and the main cause of death from cancer in Algeria **(Figure 5) [9].**

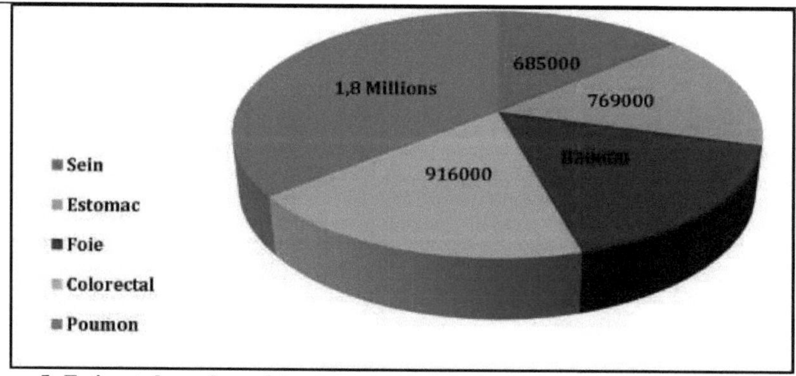

Figure 5: Estimated number of deaths from breast cancer in Algeria in 2020 [9].

Breast cancer is characterised in Algeria by the average age of women affected, which is around 35 and over, compared with 55 in developed countries. According to observations made by the President of the Algerian Association of Medical Oncology, Professor Kamel Bouzid, in a study devoted to the causes of this early-onset disease in our country, (65,000) new cases of cancer of all types have been recorded in Algeria since the beginning of 2021 until October 2021, including 15,000 cases, reported in Algiers **[11].**

Every year, Algeria records almost 50,000 new cases of all types of cancer, according to data from the national cancer register run by the National Institute of Public Health (INSP).

11.1.3. In Western Algeria

1140 female cases having undergone mastectomy were retrospectively reviewed with respect to their histoclinical and molecular characteristics. Data were collected from pathology and oncology reports from three main hospitals in western Algeria: Oran public hospital, Oran military hospital and Sidi Bel Abbes public hospital **[12].**

The exclusion criteria concerned women with a disease other than breast cancer, cases where HER2 was defined as score 2, and male breast cancer. Ethical authorisation was obtained from the hospital's ethics committee.416 new cases of breast cancer, including 151 in men and 263 in women, were identified at the Aïη Témouchent hospital **(Table I)[12].**

Table I: Distribution of breast cancer cases in Western Algeria [12].

Western Wilaya	Incidence	Year of study
ORAN	428 new cases	2020
AIN TEMOUCHENT	416 new cases (151Men/263Women)	2020
TLEMCEN	300 new cases	2018
SIDI BELABESS	214 new cases	2018

A total of 428 breast cancer patients were registered in the wilaya of Oran during the year 2020, according to the person in charge of the national breast and cervical cancer screening programme at the local Department of Health and Population (DSP**) (Mokrane F ,2020).**

Breast cancer screening, which has seen a slight decline due to the Covid-19 pandemic, has reached 4,529 women over the age of 45, she said. According to a Health and Population report, 2,397 new cases of all types of cancer were recorded in the wilaya of Oran in 2020 **[13].**

11.1.4. Epidemiology of breast cancer in young women

Breast cancer in young women is defined as cancer that occurs before the age of 35 or 40, depending on the literature. Patients diagnosed before the age of 35 account for only 2.4% of breast cancer cases, with only 1% of patients diagnosed before the age of 30 **(Chéreau E, 2019).**

Traditionally, breast cancer in young women has been associated with a more aggressive phenotype and a poorer prognosis. The relative risk of death is 39% higher in women under 40 than in older women.

(RR= 1.39 [1.34-1.35]). This risk increases by 5% for each year younger at diagnosis up to the age of 35 **[14].**

11.2 Analytical epidemiology

II.2.1 Socio-demographic factors

II.2.1.1 Age

The disease is rare in women under 30. The risk increases between the ages of 50 and 75 (almost two-thirds of breast cancers). According to the 2021 edition of the Panorama of cancers in France published by the Institut National du Cancer, 80% of breast cancers occur after the age of 50. This represents thousands of women who receive this treatment every year.

diagnosis and must combat this disease **(Figure 6) [15].**

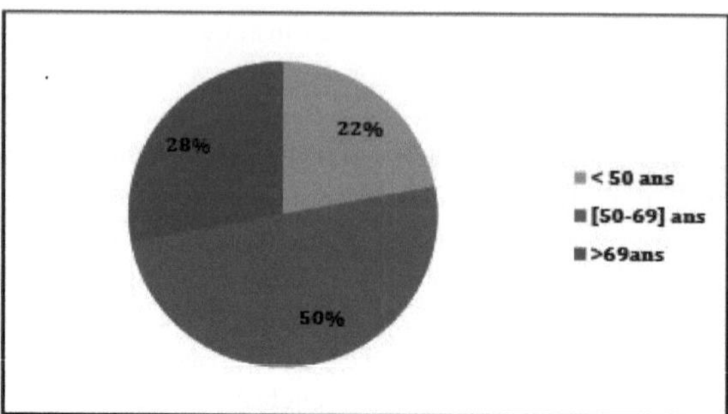

Figure 6: Incidence of breast cancer by age (2021 edition) [15].

However, this does not mean that breast cancer only affects people of a certain age. It is quite possible to develop breast cancer when you are under 40, particularly if you have a strong family history of female cancers (breast and/or ovarian) or pathogenic mutations **[15]**.

П.2.1.2 Gender

Breast cancer mainly affects women. Although it exists in men, it is 100 times less common. Men have breast tissue just like women, but their breasts are less developed. Male breast cancer is similar to female breast cancer, but there are a few differences. Male breast cancer is largely treated in the same way as breast cancer in post-menopausal women (when the ovaries have stopped producing restrogen). Less than 1% of all breast cancers affect men, and researchers estimate that by 2022 there will be 270 new cases of male breast cancer in Canada and 55 men will die from the disease **[16]**.

11.2.2 Genetic factors

It has now been established that genetics play a role in increasing the risk of certain types of breast and ovarian cancer, and that women with these conditions have genetic predispositions that increase their risk of developing breast and ovarian cancer compared with women who do not carry these genes.

Detecting the genes responsible for mutations that encourage the development of cancer is therefore a key issue in offering women with breast cancer effective, early and less burdensome treatment **[17]**.

11.2.2.1 Mutation of suppressor genes

Genetic mutations can prevent genes from working properly, causing them to become inactive. This causes cells to grow out of control, which can lead to cancer.

> **BRCA gene mutations**

It is estimated that around 2 out of every 1,000 women carry a mutation in BRCA1 or BRCA2, two genes involved in repairing the damage that DNA regularly undergoes. The presence of mutations in one of these two genes disrupts this function and greatly increases the risk of breast and ovarian cancer.

However, not all women with these genetic mutations will develop breast cancer one day, and this increases the risk of developing breast cancer at a young age, usually before the menopause. In a woman with a BRCA1 or BRCA2 mutation, the risk of breast cancer varies from 40% to 80% over the course of her life; more specifically, BRCA gene mutations increase the risk of cancer in the following way **(Figure 7) [18]**.

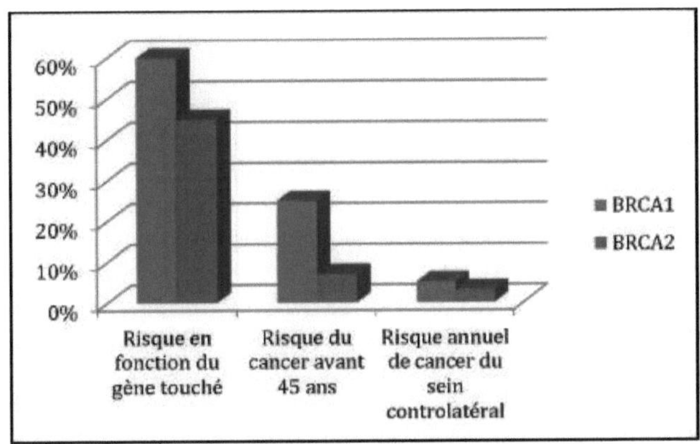

Figure 7: BRCA gene mutations increase the risk of cancer [18].

> **Mutations in the TP53 gene**

The TP53 gene is a tumour suppressor gene that controls cell growth and division. The TP53 gene also sends signals to other genes to help repair damaged DNA. If the damaged DNA cannot be repaired, the TP53 gene prevents the cell from dividing and tells it to die.

When the TP53 gene is mutated, cells with damaged DNA begin to grow and divide in a disordered fashion. Mutations in the TP53 gene are common and occur in over 50% of all cancers **[18].**

11.2.2.2 Family history, personal history and genetic inheritance

The risk of developing breast cancer also increases with family history. For example, the risk of developing breast cancer is greater if your mother or one of your mothers has had breast cancer. This risk increases further if they had their cancer before the age of 50 and if more than one of them was affected. The risk may be lower if you only have more distant relatives. However, the family history on the father's side should be considered as important as the history on the mother's side **(Figure 8) [19].**

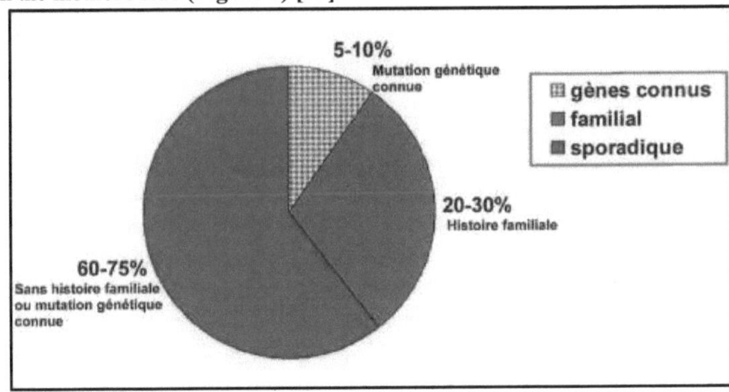

Figure 8: Family history of breast cancer (%) 2020 [19].

11.2.2.3 Precancerous lesion

Most invasive carcinomas develop from defined pre-neoplastic lesions such as atypical hyperplasia and carcinoma in situ.

11.2.3 Hygienic and dietary factors

11.2.3.1 Alcohols

According to the World Health Organisation (WHO), a simple reduction in alcohol consumption can greatly reduce the risk of cancer. Breast cancer is the most frequently diagnosed type of cancer every day, detected in 1,579 women.

Alcohol consumption is one of the main modifiable risk factors for the disease. It is responsible for 7 out of every 100 new cases of breast cancer. During "pink October", breast cancer awareness month, the WHO is encouraging everyone to understand that the risk of breast cancer can be greatly reduced simply by cutting down on alcohol consumption, which is responsible for almost 40,000 new cases of breast cancer by 2020 **[20].**

11.2.3.2 Weight gain, obesity

Breast cancer in western Algeria affects relatively young women, 34% of whom are aged under 40, with 41.11% pre-obese compared with 39.65% within normal limits and 16.62% with a BMI over 30 (obese) **(Barouagui S et *al.* , 2013).**

Obesity is associated with a hormonal profile suspected of favouring the development of breast cancer. Obesity increases the risk of breast cancer in post-menopausal women by around 50%, probably due to the increase in serum concentrations of free restradiol **(Key TJ et *al.,* 2001).**

11.2.3.3 Smoking

Smoking increases the risk of a number of cancers, including breast cancer: numerous studies have confirmed the link between smoking and breast cancer, a major risk factor that is estimated to increase the chances of developing a malignant breast tumour by 10-40%. These data have been confirmed by around 150 epidemiological studies conducted by the IARC (International Agency for Research on Cancer) since 2009**, and** it has been reported that smokers experience an early menopause and a reduced urinary concentration of restrogens. Cigarettes are a woman's worst enemy

Tobacco affects a woman's hormonal system. Because of its anti-restrogenic action, it leads to an earlier onset of the menopause. On average, smokers reach the menopause 2 years earlier than non-smokers.

Stopping smoking avoids exacerbating the symptoms (hot flushes, memory problems, etc.) **[21].**

11.2.4 Environmental factors

11.2.4.1 Ionising radiation

The effect of ionising radiation, in women exposed before the age of 40, is associated with a threefold increase in the risk of breast cancer, for an exposure evaluated at IGy**.**Over the long term, due to alterations undergone at cell level, exposure of breast tissue to ionising radiation can lead to the appearance of secondary cancers in irradiated individuals **[22].**

11.2.4.2 Exposure to certain chemicals

The 17 chemical compounds implicated include :

Aromatic amines (AA): Found in certain pharmaceutical products, plastics, rubber, glues, resins and paint dyes. **Benzene**: Found in fuel fumes, perfumes, pesticides, solvents, degreasing agents and food additives.

Butadiene: used in the manufacture of nylon, varnish, paint and synthetic rubber.

Acrylamide: In food, acrylamide is often the result of overcooking, with intense browning of food **[23].**

11.2.4.3 Electromagnetic fields

There are many sources of exposure to electromagnetic waves, from the immediate environment (radio, mobile phone), industry (welding equipment, ovens, telecommunications, radar) or medicine (magnetic resonance imaging **(Figure 9) [24].**

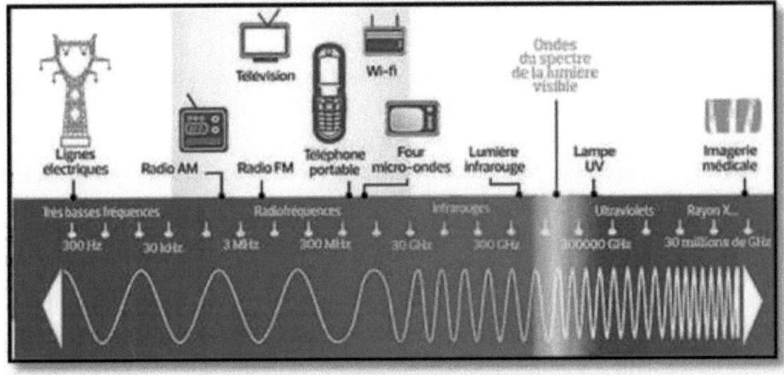

Figure 9: Electromagnetic waves [24]

The biological effects of electromagnetic fields (EMF) range from stimulation of excitable tissues (nervous system and muscles) at lower frequencies to heating of tissues at higher frequencies. Example: EBF-CEM (extremely low frequency electromagnetic fields) could be linked to an increased risk of breast cancer, particularly in pre-menopausal women **[25].**

11.2.5 Hormonal factors

11.2.5.1 Exogenous hormonal factors

> **Menopause hormone replacement therapy (HRT)**

Hormone replacement therapy (HRT) is reserved for women with an early menopause, and its effect varies according to the composition of the products. The relative risk is twofold in women using a rastroprogestogenic combination, while it is only 30% higher in women receiving rastrogen treatment alone**.** Hormone replacement therapy (HRT) is thought to have an effect on breast densification, which increases the risk of breast cancer **(Azam S et *al.* , 2018).**

> **Oral contraceptives**

They are made up of synthetic substances with effects similar to those of the hormones produced by a woman's body in preparation for pregnancy: rastrogens and progesterone. The risk of breast cancer falls as soon as consumption stops, so that 10 years after use has stopped, there is no significant increase in risk. The use of these drugs late in reproductive life leads to a relative increase in the risk of breast cancer at a time when the natural risk becomes appreciable.

Thus, the later oral contraceptives are used, the greater the number of cases of breast cancer that will result; recent use of a rastroprogestogenic pill in the previous year was associated with a 50% increased risk of breast cancer compared with women who had never taken the pill or former users **[26].**

11.2.5.2 Endogenous hormonal factors

> **Early age of first menstruation**

The average age for menarche is 12. This is the age at which, on average, a young girl

menstruates for the first time, and this increases the risk of breast cancer.
This risk is increased by early and prolonged exposure to hormonal impregnation during the active period of the ovaries. This exposure is considerable when menstrual cycles are regular. This hypothesis is consistent with the high levels of restrogens after menstruation observed in women who have menstruated early **(Key TJ et *al.*, 2001).**

> **Late menopause**

The late menopause is mainly genetic: if the mother or grandmother has experienced a late menopause, it is possible that her daughter will also experience a late menopause. Genetic causes are not systematic. Women who have their menopause after the age of 50 have an increased risk of breast cancer, compared with those whose periods stop early. The risk of breast cancer increases by around 3% for each additional year after the presumed age of menopause, known as prolonged exposure **[27].**

11.2.6 Prognostic factors

11.2.6.1 Age

Age is a prognostic factor for both local recurrence and metastatic disease. Young women under the age of 35 have a 4-fold higher risk of local recurrence than women over the age of 55 for breast cancers treated conservatively.

11.2.6.2 Stage and grade of tumour

Staging describes or classifies a cancer according to the amount of cancer present in the body and its location at the time of initial diagnosis. This is often referred to as the extent of the cancer. The information revealed by the examinations is used to determine the size of the tumour, which part of the breast is affected by the cancer, and whether the cancer has spread from its place of origin. The most commonly used staging system for breast cancer is the TNM classification, which has 5 stages: stage 0 followed by stages 1 to 4. For stages 1 to 4, the Roman numerals I, II, III and IV are often used. In general, the higher the number, the further the cancer has spread.
There are several groups of lymph nodes around each breast. The stage often depends on which lymph nodes the cancer has spread to **(Figure 10) [28].**

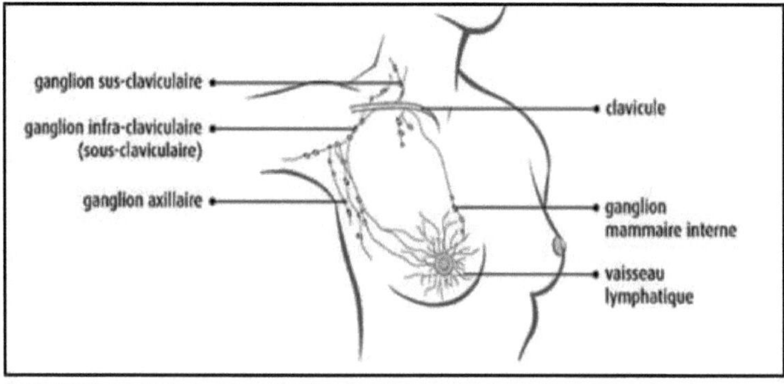

Figure 10: lymph nodes of the breast [28].

11.2.6.3 Hormone Receptor Status and HER2 Status

> **Hormone receptor status**

Hormone receptors are mainly of 2 types: restrogen receptors and progesterone receptors.

They act as a gateway for hormones to enter the cell to grow and divide. Hormone receptor status is analysed when breast cancer is diagnosed or when breast cancer recurs after treatment (recurrence) **[29].**

Hormone receptor-positive breast tumours usually have a good prognosis. They are often less aggressive, lower grade and less likely to spread than hormone receptor negative tumours. They usually respond well to hormone therapy **(Figure 11) [30].**

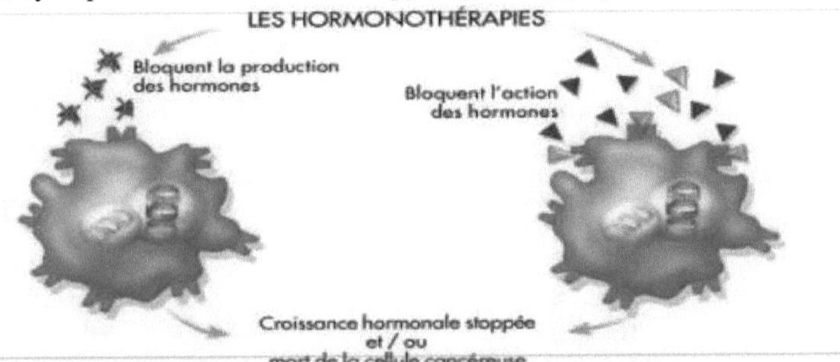

Figure 11: Effect of hormone therapy on hormone receptors [30].

In general, cancers with hormone receptors, or so-called hormone-dependent cancers, have a better outcome, and chemotherapy can be used in combination with specific hormone therapy for breast cancer.

Tests such as the Oncotype DX have been developed to assess the prognosis of the disease and can quantify the benefit of chemotherapy in patients with early-stage, HER2-negative, HR-positive breast cancer **[31].**

> **HER2 status**

Around 15% of breast cancers have an increased amount of the HER2 gene. This amplification of the gene is analysed in the cancer cells. Cancers in which the HER2 gene is over-expressed tend to behave more aggressively. However, the use of an antibody directed against HER2 (trastuzumab) has greatly improved the survival of women with this type of cancer. Other similar drugs have since been developed **[31].**

CHAPTER III

CLASSIFICATION OF THE DIFFERENT TYPES OF BREAST CANCER

III.1 TNM clinical classification

A classification known as purely "anatomical" as we currently practice it, with the "anatomical" prognostic stage which is a new prognostic classification combined more, which combines with the TNM biological tumor characteristics such as histological grade, HER2 hormone receptor status and prognostic molecular signatures and also clinical stages (AJCC, 8e edition 2017 **(Appendix III).**

III.2 Classification by histopronostic grade

Scarff, Bloom and Richardson (SBR) score modified by Elston-Ellis (Nottingham grade).

The SBR grading method consists of evaluating 3 morphological parameters: degree of differentiation (formation of tubules: glandular cavities), nuclear pleomorphism, mitotic index **(Table II), (Boughera N, 2012).**

Table II: SBR grade modified by Elston Ellis (Boughera N, 2012).

	Score 1	Score 2	Score 3
Tubulo- Glandular	>75 %	(10 -75 %)	<10%
Nuclear pleomorphism	Small, uniform cores with regular outlines	Nuclei larger than normal. Clearly visible nucleoli.	Marked pleomorphism (vesicular nuclei, prominent nucleoli)
Mitotic index	<10 mitoses	10-22	+ more than 22 mitoses

> **Total of 3 to 5:** grade I with a favourable prognosis

> **Total of 6 to 7:** grade II with intermediate prognosis

> **Total of 8 to 9:** grade III with unfavourable prognosis.

It is currently recommended that grade assessment should not be limited to invasive ductal carcinomas but should be performed for all histological subtypes for 2 main reasons: It is sometimes difficult to determine the type of tumour There may be significant morphological variations in certain histological subtypes **(Boughera N, 2012).**

III .3 Histological classification

Several types of cancer can be found in the breast, and these abnormal cells are most often located in a galactophore duct. Ductal cancer can be in situ or infiltrating, and is called intracanal or in situ carcinoma when the tumour remains confined within the duct. The cancer may also extend beyond the wall of a duct and infiltrate the breast tissue from this duct, in the case of infiltrating ductal carcinoma **[31].**

III.1.1.1 Non-invasive carcinomas (in situ)

III.1.1.1 .1 Ductal carcinoma in situ (DCIS)

They are defined as a proliferation of cytologically malignant epithelial cells confined to the interior of the galactophoric tree without invasion of the basement membrane or connective tissue. The classification of carcinoma in situ recommended by the European Pathologists' Group derives from Holland's classification and is based on nuclear grade.

> **Low-grade nuclear SCC**

Monomorphic cells with rounded nuclei, small size, few mitoses. Necrosis is rare, with intracanal proliferation of small round glandular cavities.

> **High-grade nuclear CCIS**

Pleomorphic cells, irregularly distributed, variable in size with significant atypia. The architectural type is variable, often centred by necrotic comedones.

> **Intermediate grade CCIS**

CCIS do not fall into one of the 2 previous categories **(Boughera N, 2012).**

III.1.1.2 .2 Lobular carcinoma in situ (LCIS)

This is a carcinoma of the intra-lobular ducts, which are distended and filled by a proliferation of loosely joined cells, without invasion of neighbouring connective tissue (ball sac). The cells are generally regular and small to moderate in size, with poorly stained cytoplasm and a round nucleus showing little or no mitosis.

A differential diagnosis with atypical lobular hyperplasia is necessary and this diagnosis is made with : [ductal carcinoma in situ (irregular hyperchromatic nuclei , mitoses , calcifications and necrosis)/Lobular extension of an invasive carcinoma/Atypical lobular hyperplasia]**[32].**

III.1.2.2 Invasive carcinomas

III.1.2.1 .1 Non-specific infiltrating ductal carcinoma

Tumours which do not have sufficient morphological characteristics to classify them in another category.

These tumours represent a heterogeneous group with a highly variable morphology depending on the cytological and architectural characteristics and the quantity and/or type of stroma. The tumour is nodular, firm and hard on palpation with yellowish streaks.

Prognosis: It has a 10-year survival rate of 35-50%. Prognosis is largely influenced by histological grade, tumour size, lymph node involvement and vascular emboli **(Figure 12) [33].**

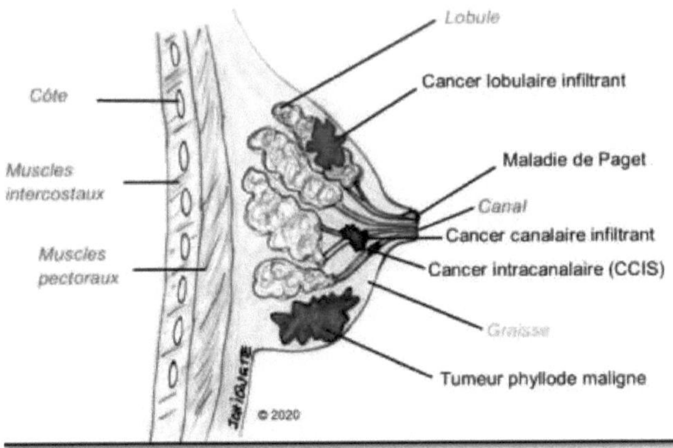

Figure 12: Different types of invasive cancer [33].

III.1.2.2 .2 Invasive lobular carcinoma (ILC) (5-15%)

An ill-defined tumour with irregular contours that originates in the lobules of the breast, then crosses these lobules and invades neighbouring breast tissue. It may also spread (metastasise) to lymph nodes and other parts of the body Architectural variations: solid or massive type, pseudo-lymphomatous, alveolar, tubulo-lobular appearance. Cellular variations: pleomorphic, kitten-ring cells **[34].**

III.1.3.3 Paget's disease of the nipple

Paget's disease of the breast is a rare type of breast cancer. It appears as a rash or other changes on the skin of the nipple, usually on one breast. It is more common in women over the age of 50 **[35].**

IV I.4 Molecular classification of breast cancer

IV.1.1 .1Basics of molecular classification

In general, breast cancers are classified into six different intrinsic subtypes, including luminal A, luminal B, HER2-enriched, normal-like basal-like and claudin-low based on the presence or absence of the three primary markers (RO, RP, and HER2), basal marker (CK5/6, EGFR) **(Pinder SE et *al.* , 2004).**

A distinction is made between tumours that express the estrogen receptor (ER+) and those that do not (ER-). The ER+ group, which is the most common, is characterised by a lesion spectrum that is essentially focused on cell proliferation. The RO- group, with a worse prognosis, includes HER2+ tumours and so-called "triple-negative" HER2- tumours. Given this multitude of profiles with different prognoses, the need to use targeted treatments has become a priority **[36].**

It was in this context that the idea emerged of classifying breast cancers according to their molecular alterations and that "molecular signatures" were born, a prognostic tool and perhaps a predictor of response to treatment. **(Franchet C et *al.* , 2015).**

The term luminal refers to the name given to one of the two cell types of normal breast tissue. These tumours are called luminal because their genes code for the proteins of the epithelial cells of the lumen of the milk ducts or lobules of the breast **(Figure 13) [36].**

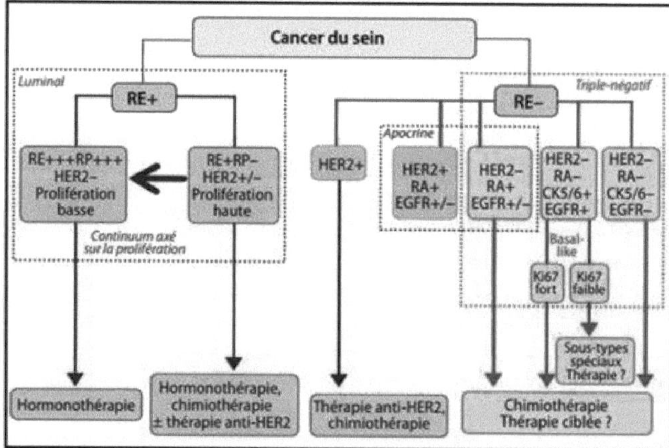

Figure 13: Classification of breast cancers and treatment decision algorithm [36].

The protein profile of these tumours is characterised by : Expression of CK8+ cytokeratins, CK18+ and CK19+Specific histological forms: lobular, mucinous, infiltrating ductal carcinoma grades I and II. A level of expression of the KI67 marker, enabling differentiation between subtypes A and B. The Ki-67 proliferation index The Ki-67 protein is associated with cell proliferation, in which increased expression of Ki-67 leads to a higher rate of cell division. Figure 1 indicates the classification of breast cancer types according to differences in immunohistochemical profile **[36].**

IV.1.2 .2 Characterisation of breast cancers by immunohistochemistry

IV.1.2.1 .1 Hormone receptors

These are proteins located on the surface of the cancer cell. They detect restrogens or progesterone passing through the bloodstream and capture them. The binding between the hormones and their receptors on the cells triggers the stimulation of the growth of these cancer cells. At present, estrogen and progesterone receptors are most often detected by immunohistochemical techniques on fixed histological sections of tumour, and more rarely by biochemical methods on frozen tumour fragments (determination by radio-ligand or fresh samples has not been carried out **[37]**.

The reliability of the immunohistochemical technique depends on a rigorous technique and compliance with certain rules. The concordance rate between hormone receptor status by immunohistochemistry and biochemistry was 86.6% for restrogen receptors (RR) and 76.8% for progesterone receptors (PR). Major discrepancies were observed in 6.3% of cases for restrogen receptors (OR) and 15.5% of cases for progesterone receptors (PR) **[37]**.

IV.1.2.2 .2 HER2 membrane receptors

HER2 is a protein naturally present in the body. It is a transmembrane receptor involved in regulating cell proliferation. When a cell becomes cancerous, the number of HER2 receptors present on its surface may increase abnormally **[37]**.

There are two techniques for testing for HER2 status: the most common is IHC (Immunohistochemistry), which is always performed first.

The result is expressed on a scale from 0 to 3+: if it is IHC 0 or 1+, the test is negative and there is no overexpression of HER2; if it is IHC 3+, the result is positive and there is overexpression of HER2. If the result is 3+, the test is positive and there is HER2 overexpression; if the result is IHC 2+, it is uncertain. The In Situ Hybridization (HIS) technique is then used to confirm or rule out HER2 overexpression. The result is either negative (HIS-) or positive (HIS+) **[38]**.

IV.1.2.3 .3 Ki67 nuclear biomarkers

Immunohistochemical detection of the Ki67 antigen has been used for many years to assess cell proliferation in cancers, but this biomarker is still not recommended for routine use in the management of breast cancers. Ki67 expression is classically detected by immunohistochemistry (IHC) in order to assess cell proliferation in tissues, and is reported in the form of a Ki67 index, which represents the percentage of labelled cells within the population studied (in cancers, this is the percentage of labelled tumour cells)**(Lacroixi and Penault , 2017).** The Ki67 index is not perfectly correlated with that of phosphorylated histone H3 (PhH3) or the mitotic index ($r = 0.79$ and $r = 0.83$, respectively), indicating that PhH3 and Ki67 provide distinct biological information and should therefore be analysed separately **(Lee LH et *al.*, 2014).**

PhH3 is a nuclear histone protein involved in chromosome condensation and cell cycle progression during mitosis and meiosis. It is a potential marker of mitotic activity, while Ki67 should be considered a marker of proliferative activity **[39]**.

V II.5 Different molecular types of breast cancer

V.1.1 .1 Luminal A subtype

It is characterised by high expression of restrogen (RO+++) and/or progesterone (PR+) hormone receptors, the absence of HER2 gene overexpression, a low level of p53 mutations and low proliferation. Tumours are often of low histological grade **[40]**.

V.1.2 .2 Luminal B subtype

It has the same characteristics with regard to hormone receptors (RO+ and/or RP+) but more often there is overexpression of the HER2+ gene. The tumours are usually of high histological grade **[40].**

V.1.3 .3 HER2 subtype (non-luminal)

When cancer cells make too many copies (overexpression) of the HER2 gene. HER2-positive breast cancer is more aggressive and more likely to spread than HER2-negative breast cancer. It is also more likely to recur after treatment. HER2+ cancer: these cancer cells have the HER2 receptor on their surface. When activated, this receptor causes cells to proliferate significantly **[40].**

V.1.4 .4 Triple negative sub-type

When no restrogen receptor, no progesterone receptor and no trace of HER2 are found in a cancer, it is called a triple-negative cancer.

CHAPTER IV

TRIPLE-NEGATIVE BREAST CANCER

VI .1 Definition

Triple-negative breast cancer is known as a heterogeneous type of cancer that is classified into six subtypes. The subtypes are immunomodulatory (IM), luminal androgen receptor (LAR), basal-like 1 (BL-1), basal-like 2 (BL-2), mesenchymal (M) and mesenchymal stem-like (MSL).It is associated with a younger age at diagnosis. Its main risk factor is a mutation in the BRCA1 and BRCA2 genes. These mutations are found in around 30% of cases. On the positive side, this genetic component opens the way to new therapeutic approaches, such as PARP inhibitor drugs **[41]**.

VII2 Epidemiology of triple-negative breast cancer

I.5.2.1 Epidemiology of triple-negative breast cancer in young women in western Algeria

According to various studies, the incidence of triple-negative breast cancer varies between 12 and 20% of all breast cancers. In our country, **(Cherbal F et *al.*, 2015)** presented an initial original study on the epidemiology of triple-negative breast cancer in Algerian patients. The study was carried out on 3,403 breast cancer patients and identified 737 cases of triple-negative breast cancer; the proportion of triple-negative breast cancer was therefore estimated at 21.65%, affecting more young women with an average age at diagnosis of 46 years **(Cherbal F et *al.*, 2015).**

I.5.1 Main characteristics of triple-negative breast cancer

Triple-negative breast cancer represents a very aggressive group of tumours, and this aggressiveness is undoubtedly due to the very specific characteristics of this molecular subtype **(Appendix IV) [42].**

One of the explanations for the poor prognosis of triple-negative breast cancers undoubtedly lies in their particular evolutionary profile, with a high rate of proliferation, a high nuclear grade, a greater susceptibility to metastasis, and the low or high expression of certain molecules **(Reis F et *al.* , 2008)**.

I.5.2 Specific classification of triple-negative breast cancer

The first is the standard specific DNA microarray technique developed by Parker in 2009 called PAM50 to analyse the gene expression profile of breast cancer tumours.

PAM50 (Prediction Algorithm of Microarray 50) analyses the expression profile of a series of 50 genes in breast cancer tumours using the microarray technique combined with RT-qPCR.

Cluster analysis enabled this interesting study to identify 6 transcriptomic subtypes, with different gene profiles, biology and sensitivity to treatments **(Prat et *al.* , 2010)**:

1.5.4.1 Basal-like subtype 1(BL-1)

Representing 10% of triple-negative breast cancers, it is characterised by the expression of cell cycle and DNA damage response genes.

1.5.4.2 Basal-like subtype 2(BL-2)

Represents 20% of triple-negative breast cancers and shares with basal like 1 (BL1) part of the cell cycle genes, also contains genes from the signalling pathway of the growth factor receptor family, as well as the expression of myoepithelial markers.

1.5.4.3 Immunomodulators (IM) subtype

Accounts for 20% of triple-negative breast cancers and expresses genes involved in immune signalling **[42].**

1.5.4.4 Mesenchymal-like(ML) subtype

Accounts for 20% of triple-negative breast cancers and is enriched in genes regulating cell motility, invasion and mesenchymal differentiation **[43].**

1.5.4.5 Mesenchymal stem-like (MSL) subtype

Representing 10% of triple-negative breast cancers, it is enriched in genes regulating epithelial-mesenchymal transformation, cancer stem cell pathways and angiogenesis **[43].**

I.5.3 Triple-negative breast cancer and BRCA breast cancer predisposition genes

1.5.5.1 BRCA1 gene and protein

The BRCA1 gene is located in the q21 region between markers D17s1321 and D17s1325 on chromosome 17. It is a very large gene covering 80 kb of genomic DNA. Its coding sequence comprises 5589 base pairs and is made up of 24 exons, including two non-coding exons, exon 1 and 4 **(Figure 14) [44].**

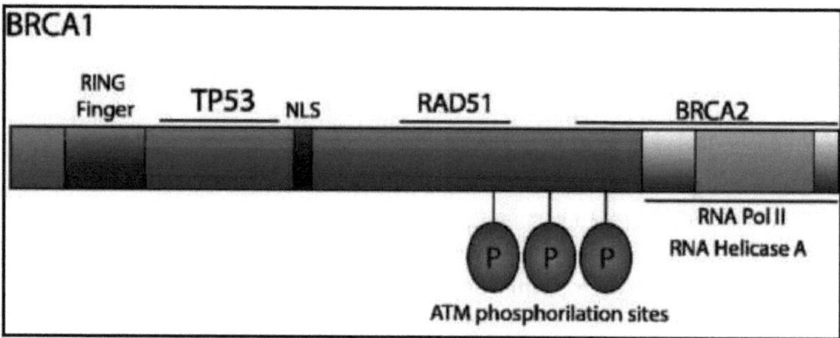

Figure 14: Structure of the BRCA1 gene [44].

Transcription of the BRCA1 gene leads to the synthesis of a ubiquitous 7.8 kb mRNA. The most common BRCA1 transcript codes for a complex nuclear protein of 1863 amino acids and 220 kDa molecular weight, the level of which depends on the cell cycle. It has numerous functional domains which interact with more than 20 proteins and have different functions **(Figure 15) [44].**

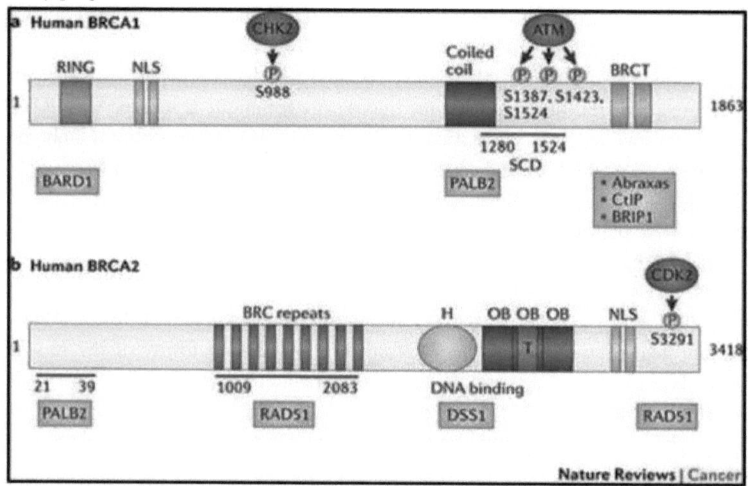

Figure 15: Functional domains of BRCA1 and BRCA2 proteins [44].

> **Two BRCT domains (BRCA1 Carboxyl-Terminus)**

In its carboxy-terminal part, which is a tandem of two homologous motifs comprising 110 amino acids. These domains are common to several proteins involved in DNA repair **(Boulton SJ , 2006).**

> **A RING FINGER domain**

Located N-terminally, it is a catalytic domain involved in ubiquitination and protein-protein and protein-DNA interaction. Allowing interactions with other proteins including BARD1.on has a zinc domain, it has been identified as a nuclear export sequence (NES), necessary for export of the protein to the cytoplasm, which opposes the two nuclear localisation signals (NLS: Nuclear Localization Signal) present in the 5' part of exon 11, essential for nuclear localisation of the BRCA1 protein **(Chen CF et *al.* , 1996).**

1.5.5.2 BRCA 2 gene and BRCA 2 protein

Following the cloning of the BRCA1 gene, the second breast cancer susceptibility gene, named BRCA2, was very quickly located on the long arm of chromosome 13, then identified by positional cloning of the 13q12-q13 chromosomal region between markers D13S289 and D13S267 **(Wooster R et *al.*, 1994).**

BRCA2 is a large gene spread over 84 kb of genomic DNA, with a length of 10,257 bp. It consists of 27 exons (exon 1 is not coding), the majority of which are small, except for two large central exons (exon 10:1116bp and exon 11:4932bp), representing 59% of the coding part, and 48% for exon 11 alone. Introns account for 86% of the genomic sequence **(Figure 16) [44].**

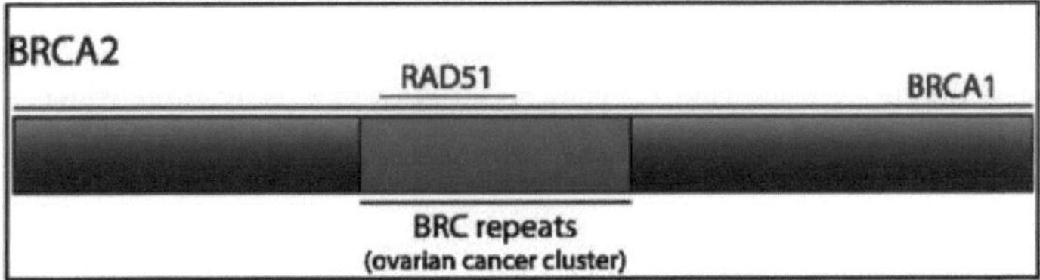

BRC repeats (ovarian cancer cluster)

Figure 16: Structure of the BRCA2 gene [44].

The 26 exons of the BRCA2 gene are transcribed into a messenger RNA of almost 11,386 bp (this is the most frequent transcript), translated into one of the largest polypeptides in the human proteome, consisting of 3,418 amino acids (380 kDa).Several functional domains have been identified in the BRCA2 protein **(Figure 15)[44] :**

> **BRCs repeat domain**

Repeated eight times over 1000 amino acids in exon 11, each BRC domain is composed of around 70 amino acids and is conserved in several mammalian species, suggesting a primordial function **[45].**

> **Area C- terminal**

In addition to the BRC domains, a second binding site for the RAD51 protein is present at the C-terminus (this site contains Serine3291 which, depending on its phosphorylation state by Cdk (cyclindependent kinase), modulates the binding of RAD51 to it **(Esashi F et *al.* , 2005).**

> **DNA-binding domain**

It contains 5 distinct domains in the carboxy-terminal part. The first domain is a helical domain that binds to the DSS1 polypeptide.

> **Domain N terminal**

Which interacts with the PALB2 protein, the conserved peptide sequence encoded by the third exon of BRCA2, is thought to have the capacity to activate transcription **(Esashi F et *al.* , 2005).**

1.5.5.3Functional role of the two proteins BRCA1 and BRCA 2

> **Detection, signalling and repair of DNA damage**

Homologous recombination (HR) is considered to be the most reliable pathway, and therefore comes into play in the S and G2 phases of the cell cycle. BRCA1 functions mainly as a mediator between breakage detection proteins and repair proteins. In addition, some studies suggest that BRCA1 is also involved in non-homologous end joining (NHEJ) repair. BRCA2, for its part, is only involved in the HR repair pathway, through interaction with and regulation of the RAD51 recombinase, thus ensuring its localisation and function at sites of DNA damage **(Henderson ,2012).**

> **Regulation of transcription**

BRCA1 is involved in the basic transcriptional machinery by interacting with the RNA polymerase II complex via RNA helicase A. **Several transcription factors (both co-repressors and co-activators) interact with BRCA1, including p53, ESR1 and CtIP.** Several transcription factors (both co-repressors and co-activators) interact with BRCA1, including p53, ESR1 and CtIP.BRCA1 has also been associated with repression of ER-α signalling, which causes restrogen-induced inhibition of cell growth **[45].**

1.5.5.4Molecular pathology of the BRCA 1 AND BRCA 2 genes

Inactivation of the BRCA1 and BRCA2 genes is a source of genetic errors which, when they accumulate, can lead to genomic instability. Individuals carrying pathogenic mutations are particularly at risk of developing breast and ovarian cancers. Complete inactivation of the BRCA1 and BRCA2 genes by biallelic mutations in individuals often results in a lethal phenotype. However, germline mutations in BRCA1 and BRCA2 explain only about 25% of breast cancer cases, with BRCA1 accounting for about 15% of hereditary breast cancers and about 45% of hereditary breast and ovarian cancers **[46].**

1.5.5.5Metastases from triple-negative breast cancer

Cancer begins with the development of cancer cells. These cells multiply and form a tumour. The more the cells multiply, the bigger the tumour becomes. There is then a risk of cancer cells escaping from the tumour and colonising neighbouring organs or other parts of the body. These "secondary" cancers are called metastases **[47].**

Several studies have demonstrated the very early and aggressive nature of the metastatic spread of triple-negative breast cancer (TNBC), with a tendency for synchronous visceral metastases and a greater risk of metastatic recurrence in the first 5 years **(Liedtke C et *al.* , 2008).**

CHAPTER V

THERAPEUTIC STRATEGIES

V .1 Surgery

For "T1" tumours, conservative surgery (lumpectomy) may sometimes be recommended for "T2" tumours. For larger multifocal or multicentric tumours, a mastectomy should be performed. If the form occurs in the presence of a BRCA1 mutation, total mastectomy may be proposed, possibly as contralateral prophylaxis. Adjuvant treatment with radiotherapy and chemotherapy will be administered after surgery. The prognosis for triple-negative breast cancer is less favourable than for other forms, with a risk of invasive recurrence. Most of these recurrences occur within three years of surgery, but the risk diminishes rapidly thereafter **[48].**

V .2 Chemotherapy

Chemotherapy is effective for so-called chemosensitive cancers, generally consisting of 4 cycles of AC (Adriamycin (A)/cyclophosphamide (C)) 60mg, or Epirubicin 90 mg Cyclophosphamide 600 mg (E90C600) every 14 days followed by 12 weekly infusions of paclitaxel 80 mg. Chemotherapy may be neoadjuvant, adjuvant or used to treat advanced stages of the disease **[48].**

V .3 Cytotoxic chemotherapy

Cytotoxic chemotherapy is the only approved treatment for triple-negative breast cancer. More than 80% of women with this type of breast cancer are treated with chemotherapy including anthracyclines, which can cause serious cardiotoxic side-effects. To date, in the absence of molecularly targeted therapies, cytotoxic chemotherapy remains the keystone of treatment in neoadjuvant, adjuvant and metastatic settings, and the only systemic treatment currently validated **(Goldhirsch A et *al.* , 2011)**.

Because of their specificity in causing irreversible double-stranded DNA damage, particularly in the case of BRCA gene deficiency, they can subsequently promote tumour cell apoptosis **[49].**

V .4 Targeted therapy

Targeted therapies are among the new weapons that have joined the therapeutic arsenal dedicated to the fight against breast cancer, alongside traditional chemotherapy, radiotherapy, hormone therapy and mastectomy or lumpectomy **[50].**There is a wide variety of targeted therapies, designed to act on different tumour characteristics:

V.4.1 Trastuzumab, Herceptin

It is a monoclonal antibody, a drug that targets the HER2 protein, a growth factor that stimulates the proliferation of cancer cells.

It is estimated that 12% to 20% of breast cancers 'overexpress' this protein, i.e. they have a high level of it. By intercepting the binding between HER2 and cancer cells, trastuzumab slows or stops cell division **(Figure 17) [51].**

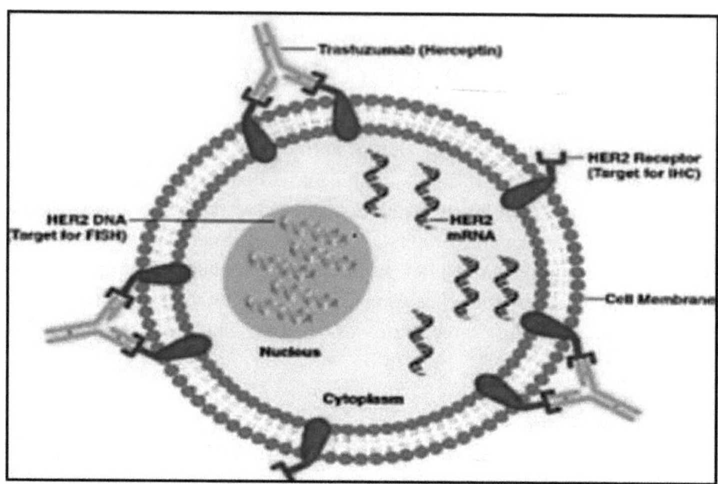

Figure 17: Mechanism of the monoclonal antibody Trastuzumab [51].

V.4.2 Bevacizumab, or Avastin

It is another monoclonal antibody and an anti-angiogenic, targeting the VEGF (Vascular Endothelial Growth Factor) protein. This stimulates the growth of blood vessels. This drug prevents cancer cells from developing the blood supply they need for oxygenation and nutrient intake, thereby slowing tumour growth.

It binds to VEGF, a key factor in vasculogenesis and angiogenesis, thereby inhibiting the binding of VEGF to its receptors, Flt-1 (VEGFR-1) and KDR (VEGFR-2), on the surface of endothelial cells.

Neutralising the biological activity of VEGF causes tumour vessels to regress, normalises the remaining tumour vessels and inhibits the formation of new tumour vessels, thereby inhibiting tumour growth **(Figure 18) [52].**

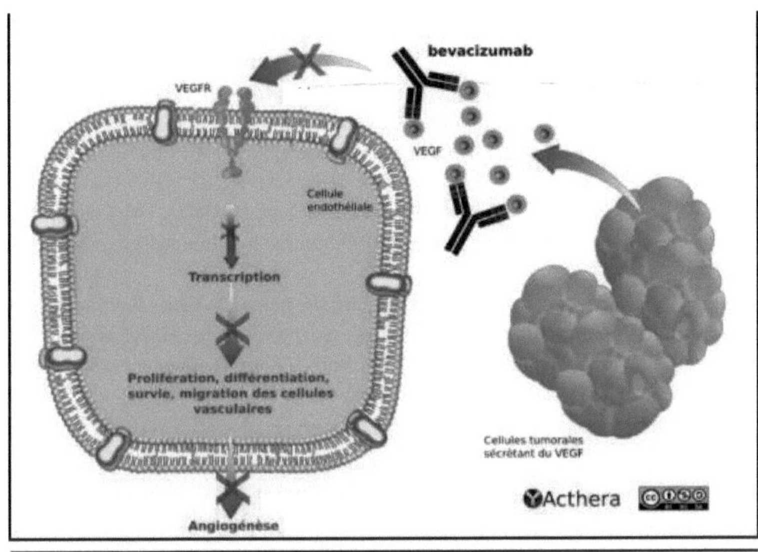

Figure 18: Mechanism of action of Bevacizumab [52].

V.4.3 Lapatinib (Tyverb) and everolimus (Afinitor)

Are inhibitors of the intracellular domains of EGFR (ErbB1) and HER2 (ErbB2) receptor protein kinases, with low dissociation from these receptors (half-life greater than or equal to 300 minutes) proteins involved in cell growth. These drugs bind to cancer cells to stop cell division and limit their proliferation **[53].**

Lapatinib (4-anilino-quinazoline) inhibits ErbB receptor-dependent tumour cell growth *in vitro* and in several animal species. The growth inhibitory effect of lapatinib was tested on cell lines conditioned with trastuzumab. *In vitro*, it maintained significant activity on breast tumour cell lines selected for long-term growth on a medium containing trastuzumab **(Figure 19) [54].**

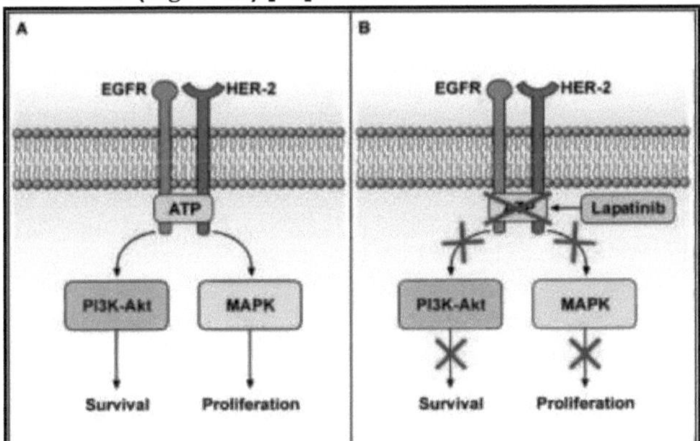

Figure 19 Mechanisms of resistance to Lapatinib in HER2-induced breast cancer [54].

Triple-negative" breast cancers are treated with chemotherapy, surgery, radiotherapy and

immunotherapy. The patient will receive neither hormonal treatment nor targeted anti-HER2 therapy.
In the case of a BRCA1 or BRCA2 gene mutation, treatment with a PARP inhibitor may be proposed. Cells with a dysfunction of the BRCA-1 pathway would also be sensitive to inhibitors of an enzyme, poly (ADP-ribose) polymerase (PARP). In these BRCA-1 deficient tumours, DNA break repair is impossible if both the PARP and HR (homologous recombination) repair pathways are inhibited. However, loss of BRCA-1 function inhibits the HR pathway and tumour cells subjected to PARP inhibitors are doomed to apoptosis **(Freres P et al. , 2010).**
Triple-negative breast cancers are so named because the cells that make them up overexpress neither the restrogen receptor, nor the progesterone receptor, nor the HER2 biomarker. These three proteins are the targets of the most effective anti-tumour treatments currently available. Targeted therapies can act at different levels of the cell:

> On growth factors (which are messengers that trigger the transmission of information within a cell).

> On their receptors (which enable information to be transferred within the cell).

> On elements inside the cells **[55].**

CHAPTER VI

MATERIALS & METHODS

In order to carry out and deepen our study, I carried out a practical training period in the anatomopathology laboratory of the University Hospital Establishment of Oran "1st November 1954" (EHUO) from 29 January to 02 March 2022.

VI.1 Population studied

This is a retrospective and prospective study of the last six years from 2017 to 2022 involving a sample of 480 patients diagnosed and operated on at the Etablissement Hôspitalier Universitaire d'Oran (EHUO) "1er Novembre 1954". Samples were recruited from the infiltrating ductal carcinoma (IDC) and infiltrating lobular carcinoma (ILC) tumour blocks. Of these samples, only 59 patients met the criteria for our present study. The latter are triple-negatives, a group of tumours characterised by the absence of hormone receptors (progesterone, restrogen) and HER2 protein on the surface of their cells. They are therefore ineligible for treatments targeting all three types of marker.

Our samples are subdivided into three histological types such as :

51 patients with invasive ductal carcinoma (IDC), 6 patients with invasive lobular carcinoma (ILC) and 2 patients with both histological types of invasive carcinoma (lobular and ductal).

VI.2 Conduct of the study

To carry out this work, I obtained data from the medical records of patients included by informed consent, using a data processing form (standardised medical questionnaire) **(Appendix I).** The clinicopathological parameters are shown in the summary table **(Table XXXVI) (Appendix VII).**

The data used are included in the extracted table **(Table XXXV) (Appendix VI).** All the parameters meet our criteria for this study.

VI.3 Working methods

Anatomopathological methods are based on macroscopic and microscopic examination of cell preparations (cytopathology) or tissue preparations (histopathology). The analysis of our samples is divided into three main areas:

- Standard histological study.
- Immunohistochemical study.

VI.3.1 Classical histological study

Histological analysis of breast lesions involves the microscopic reading of tissue (taken by the surgeon or radiologist) by a pathologist specialised in reading breast samples. His expertise is extremely important in all treatment decisions. When a sample arrives at the laboratory, it is registered and given a unique identification number, which is transcribed onto the blocks and slides.

VI.3.1.1 Fixing

After sampling and microscopy, which allows the general appearance of the specimen to be observed, the specimen must be fixed to prevent degradation. Fixing the samples Place the samples in a tissue fixative as quickly as possible.

Delayed or poor fixation reduces the morphological quality of the histological sections, while respecting the ratio between the quantity of tissue and the volume of fixative (1:10).

Open the surgical parts to allow adequate penetration of the tissue (cut the mammectomies into booklets, keeping the skin intact). Isolate the tumour nodule and fix it separately, then isolate the axillary curage and the nipple). Fixation times vary according to the fixative used and the volume of the part to be fixed. The optimum fixation times vary according to the fixative used; they are 24 hours for partial breast exeresis and 48 hours for mastectomies fixed in buffered formalin **(Figure 20).**

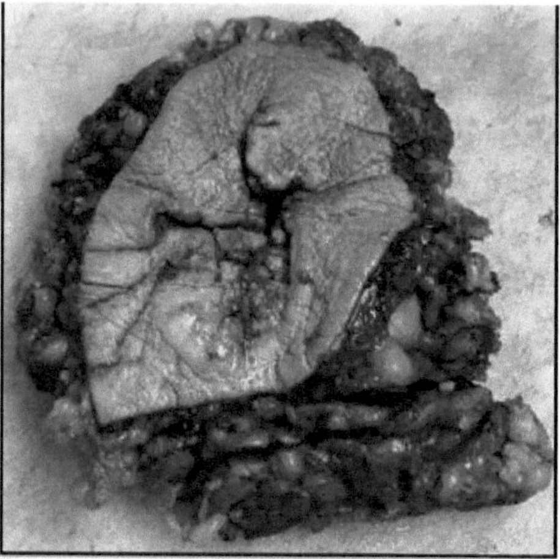

Figure 20: Mastectomy of very advanced right breast fixed in 10% formalin (personal photo)

VI.3.1.2 Macroscopic study

The detailed macroscopic examination is an essential part of the study of a surgical specimen. The specimen is examined, measured, weighed, palpated and then dissected using a scalpel; we will take this left mastectomy specimen covered with a skin flap as an example **(Figure 21).**

The samples (contained in the cassettes) are then fixed overnight in formaldehyde. Formaldehyde is a fast-penetrating, slow-fixing chemical that is best suited to large pieces of tissue, and reacts with the side chains of proteins to form hydroxy-methyl groups. The effects of formaldehyde are reversible with excess water. This allows morphological conservation of tissue and cell structures.

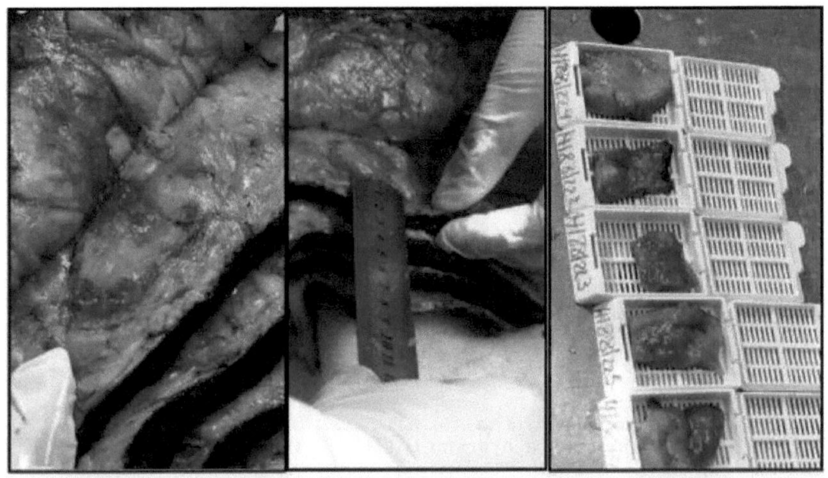

Figure 21 Macroscopic study of a breast operative specimen (personal photo)

VI.3.1.3 Dehydration

After arranging the cassettes, we move on to the hydration stage using an automatic machine **(Figure 22),** which contains 12 tanks for the gradual dehydration of the samples, increasing alcohols up to 100% (dehydration) **(Table III)** because paraffin is immiscible in water, then a solvent such as xylene, which is known as the substitution stage for clarification, then hot paraffin (liquid) for impregnation.

These transfers can be automated. The duration of the various stages varies according to the type of tissue to be included.

Table III: Dehydration and substitution protocol.

Bins	Duration
2 B formaldehyde	1h30m each
1 B 70% alcohol	2h
1 B 80% alcohol	2h
2 B alcohol 96	2 hours each
2 B 100% alcohol	2 hours each
2 B of Xylene	2 hours each
2 B of paraffin	2 hours each

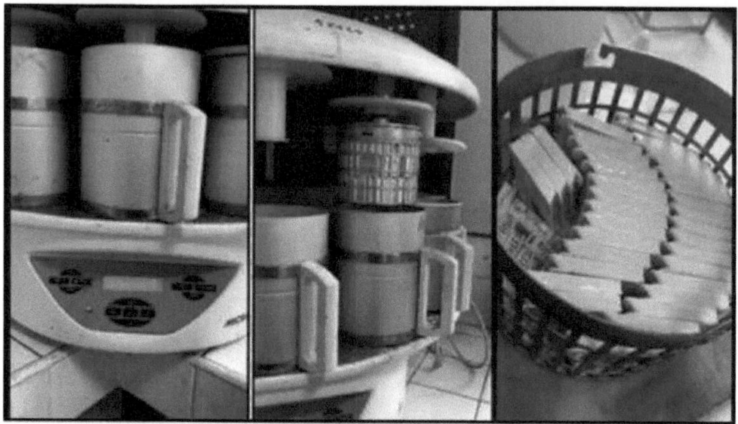

Figure 22: Automatic dehydrator (LEICA TP1020) (personal photo)

VI.3.1. 4Inclusion

The parts are placed in a metal mould filled with paraffin (hot and therefore liquid at 70°C), associated with a support (bearing the identification number).

The whole assembly is then cooled to solidify the paraffin in a block or on a cold plate, otherwise it is placed directly in the freezer (**-54°C) (Figure 23).** Once solidified, the block is removed from the mould,

the part is caught in the block.

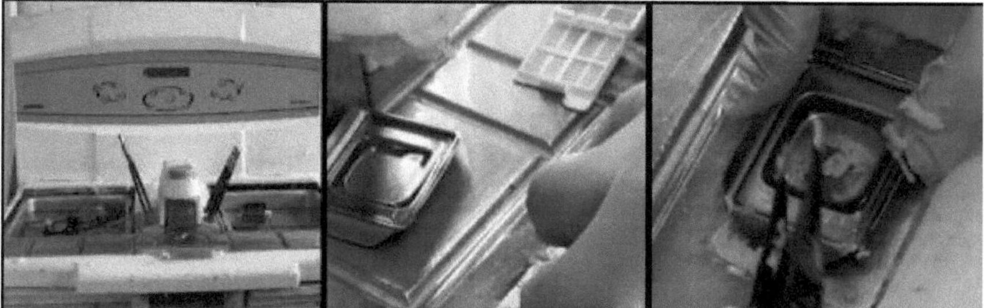

Figure 23: Inclusion of mastectomy samples (personal photo)

VI.3.1.5 Microtome sections

Before using the microtome, the block must first be cleaned and deburred so that it can be hung properly later. The microtome allows the block to be cut to a thickness of 1 to 4 µm, allowing the microscope's light rays to pass through and avoiding cellular superimposition.

The result is a very fragile ribbon that must be treated with care **(Figure 24).**

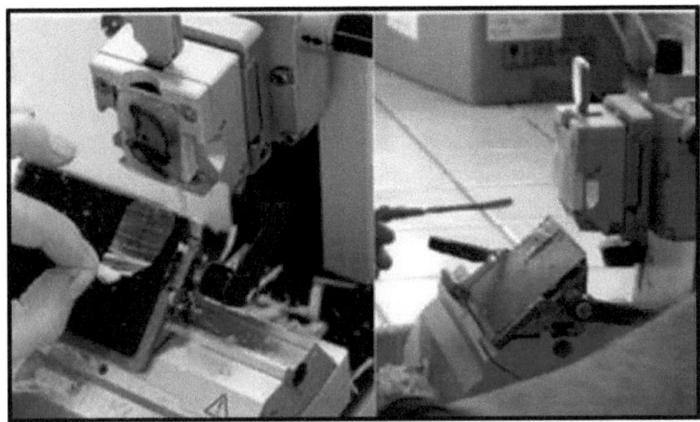

Figure 24: Cutting on the manually-rotated Leica microtome (personal photo)

Histocore Biocut - Manual rotation microtome: This is one of the most ergonomic microtomes on the market, allowing us to quickly and efficiently select the most comfortable direction of rotation with the approximate customised feed wheel.

Once the slides have been spread out and heated, they are labelled with the patient and block number written in pencil **(Figure 25).** The next step is deparaffinisation, which consists of removing the paraffin surrounding the fragment by placing the dry slides in small trolleys in an oven at 37°C for approximately 24 hours **(Figure 26).**

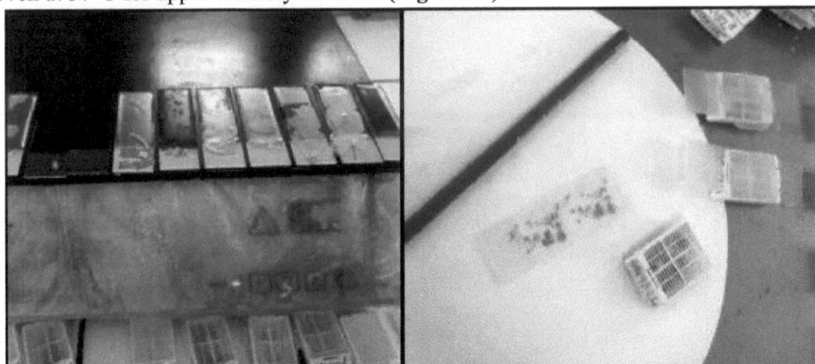

Figure 25: Spreading the ribbons on the slides (personal photo)

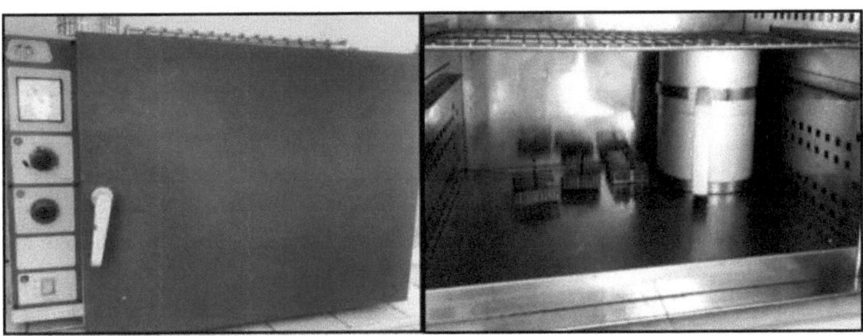

Figure 26: Dewaxing in the oven (personal photo)

VI.3.1.6 Colouring

Histological staining is used to highlight important characteristics of the tissue, as well as to differentiate structural elements of the tissue by their colour or the intensity of their staining. At the technology platform, the basic staining of slides is done with haematoxylin-eosin.

It produces a complete image of the microanatomy of a tissue and is frequently used by pathologists and researchers as an initial assessment.

The usual stain combines a nuclear basic dye (haematein, haematoxylin) and a cytoplasmic acid dye (eosin, erythrosin or phloxin).Ématoxylin-eosin combines haematein, which stains nuclei purple, and eosin, which stains cytoplasm pink. After dewaxing, the cells are passed through 12 staining trays using stainless steel racks (**Table IV**) **(Figure 27).**

Table IV: Steps in the classical histology technique

Baths	Duration
3 toluene or xylene baths	5 min in each bath
2 alcohols	5 min in each bath
rinse	Distilled water
Haematoxylin	5 minutes
Rinsing in acidified water	3.4.5 dives
Lithium carbonate rinse	3.4.5 Diving
Alcohol rinse	2 min
Iosine	3.4.5 Diving
3 acetone baths	5 min in each bath
toluene	5 min and more.

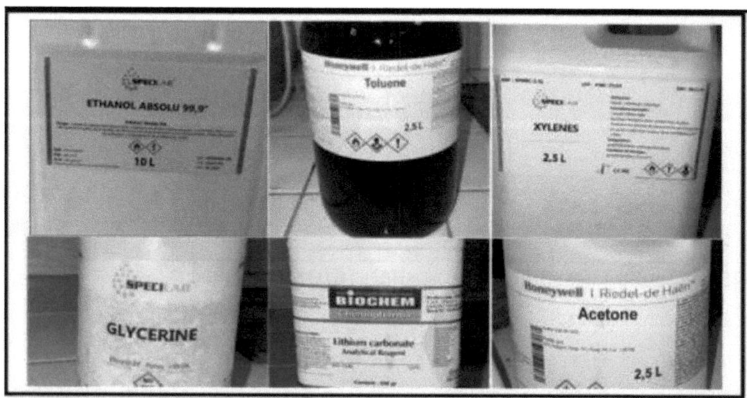

Figure 27: Products used for Haematoxylin and Eosin staining (personal photos)

VI.3.1.7 Assembly

The cuts are mounted between slides and lamellae with a product (EuKitt) containing 45% acrylic resin and 55% xylene. Dries quickly (20min) without forming air bubbles and remains optically clear for over 10 years. Refractive index close to that of glass, allowing them to adhere. The slides are ready for storage or observation **(Figure 28).**

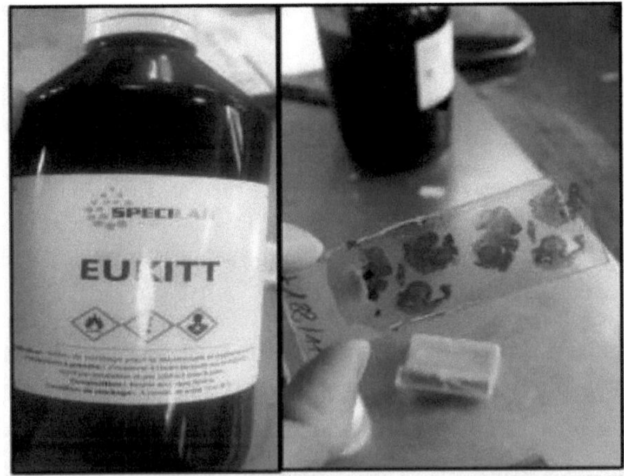

Figure 28: Mounting the slides using glue (acrylic and xylene resin) (personal photo)

VI.3.2 Immunohistochemical study

Immunohistochemistry is an additional test used to clarify a diagnosis and to better classify a tumour (malignancy, benignity, tumour classification).

Our antibody panel (the Autostainer Link 48) is combined with revolutionary software and connectivity options, offering an exceptional level of integration that delivers high productivity and efficient workflow. The Autostainer Link 48 guarantees optimal staining results and offers a large capacity for slides and reagents. Save space and centralise slide programming and we can diagnose a wide range of tumour types **(Figure 29)**.

This is a method for detecting proteins or other antigens in tissue sections. To do this, the sections are exposed to labelled antibodies directed against epitopes of the target protein.

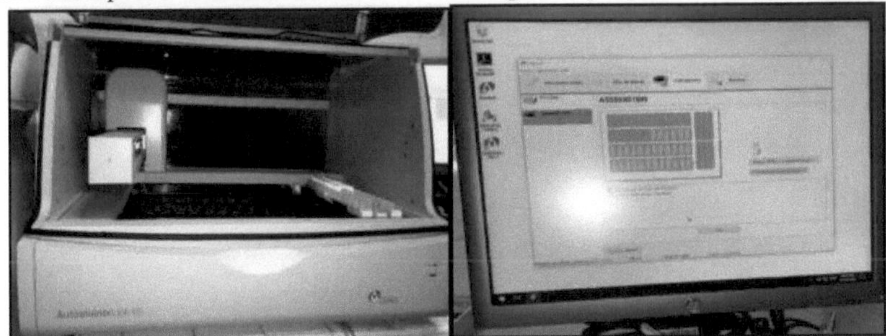

Figure 29: DaKo Autostamer Link 48 immunohistochemistry system (personal photo)

It is then possible to visualise a target using a marker, for example a fluorescent dye, an enzyme, a radioactive tracer or colloidal gold. Antibodies can be applied in two distinct ways: directly, by binding a label-conjugated antibody to its target substance, or indirectly, by incubating the primary antibody in the target substance and then binding a labelled secondary antibody to the primary antibody.

There are five main stages in this technique:

- Dewaxing.

- Antigen unmasking.
- Enzyme blocking (endogenous peroxidase).
- Deposition of primary and secondary antibodies.
- Mayer haematoxylin counterstain and slide mounting.

11.3.1.1 Dewaxing :

Incubate the slides in an oven at 17°C for 24 hours, then pass the section through 3 xylene baths for 5 minutes each. Wash the section in 96%, 80% and 70% benzyl alcohol baths for 5 minutes each, then rinse with distilled water (30 seconds) to dewax, dehydrate and clean the tissue.

11.3.1.2 Unmasking

Endogenous peroxidases are blocked by incubating the tissue in 3% hydrogen peroxide (H2O2) for 10 min. Rinsed with distilled water, the samples are then unmasked by the antigen.

First immerse the slide in Tris-EDTA buffer, pH 9.0, 0.05%Tween- 20 *† , and incubate at 95°C in a water bath for 30 minutes. Remove the slide at room temperature and allow to cool in Tris-EDTA buffer, pH 9.0 for 15 min. Rinse with distilled water. Wash in 0.05 M Tris-HCL buffer (pH 7.6) with 0.2% Tween-20 (Buffer A) for 5 minutes.

11.3.1.3 Enzyme blocking

The blocking of endogenous peroxidases is a necessary step in immunohistochemical analysis with horseradish peroxidase labelling. If this step is omitted from the protocol, endogenous peroxidases can cause precipitation of chromogens, resulting in background staining.

The sample is circled and 3 drops of 3% hydrogen peroxide (H2O2) solution are added for 5 min to promote antigen/antibody complexes. The slides are then placed in a bath containing PBS (Phosphate Buffered Saline) wash buffer for one hour.

minute **(Figure 30).**

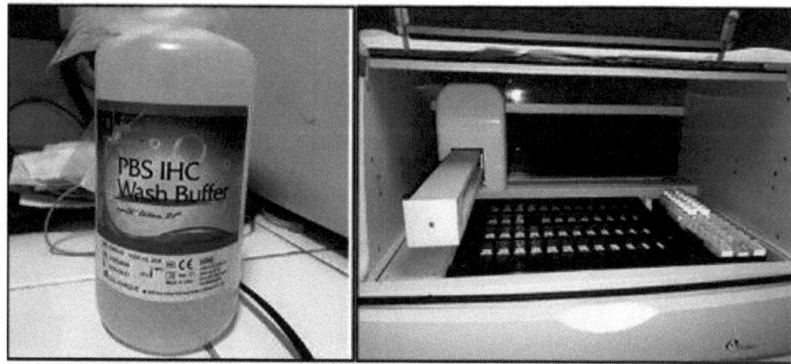

Figure 30:,washing with PBS buffer (personal photo)

II.3.1.4 Application of antibodies

*** Application of the primary antibody**

The primary antibody (Anti RE , Anti RP ,Anti HER2 or Anti Ki67) (according to the labels on the slides diluted in 0.05 M Tris-HCL buffer (pH 7.6) with 0.05% Tween- 20 at a dilution of between 1/100 and 1/200 is applied to the tissue for 1 hour in a humid chamber using an automatic pipette, then rinsed twice for 5 minutes in PBS.

- Application of the secondary antibody

Put 2 drops of Biotinylated secondary antibody on the tissue and leave to incubate for 15 min. Then rinse with PBS to apply the standard immunohistochemistry protocol (HRP - Peroxide - DAB), washing twice for 5 minutes in the buffer **(Figure 31)**.

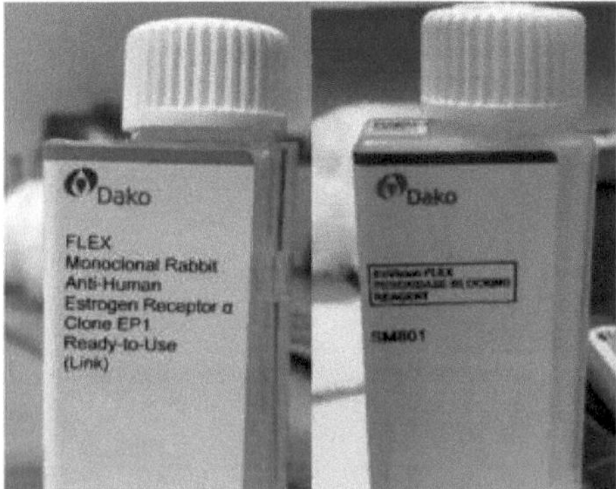

Figure 31: Primary antibodies (RE, HER2) used in iininunoliistocliinia (personal photo)

11.3.1.5 Revelation of peroxidase activity

For better sensitivity and contrast, apply 2 drops of chromogen (Diaminobenzidine) (chromogen which reacts with peroxidase in the presence of hydrogen peroxide to give a coloured product visible under an optical microscope), protect the slides from light with a solution prepared in advance and leave on the slides for 10 min, rinse 3 times at 2 min with distilled water.

11.3.1.6 Haematoxylin counterstaining

Counterstaining is carried out with Mayer's haematoxylin, which stains the nuclei intensely purplish blue, as well as the cytoplasm. The slides are immersed for 5 min, then dipped in a 2% ammonia water bath, followed by immersion in alcohol for 1 min, then xylene for 1 min.

11.3.1.7 Mounting the lanes

The coverslips are mounted on the slides using EuKitt or aqueous Paramount (**Figure 32**).

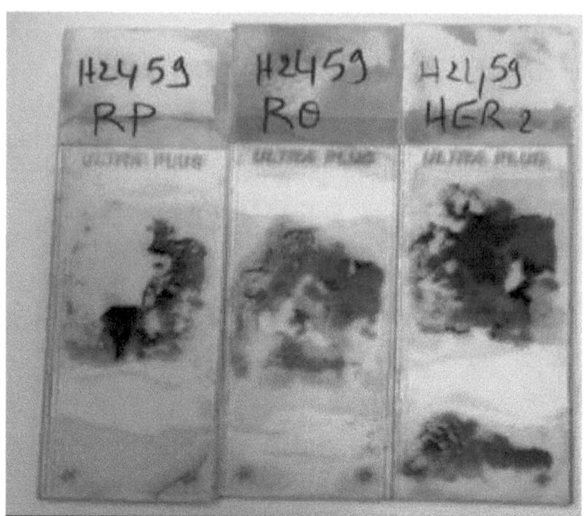

Figure 32: Assembly of slides stained with Mayer's haematoxylin (personal photo)

VI .4 Statistical analysis

Statistical data were analysed using IBM SPSS 21 software. The Chi2 test was used to compare percentages with statistical significance defined at $p < 0.05$.

CHAPTER VII

RESULTS

We conducted a retrospective and prospective study of 59 patients with triple-negative breast cancer, whose tumours were of the histological types infiltrating ductal carcinoma (IDC) and lobular carcinoma. The latter were classified by immunohistochemical method. The results are subdivided into three sections: qualitative results, descriptive results and analytical results.

VII.1 Qualitative results

VII.1.1 Results of the histological study using haematoxylin and eosin staining

Histopathological examination using a light microscope (Leica) enabled us to identify the main histological type of our samples: infiltrating ductal carcinoma, the most frequent and variable form of malignant breast tumours. We will take as an example the patient (H2494) with a histological aspect of a non-specific infiltrating carcinoma of the right breast, with a PTNM stage (AJCC 8th edition 2017) (T2N1a), **(Figure 33).**

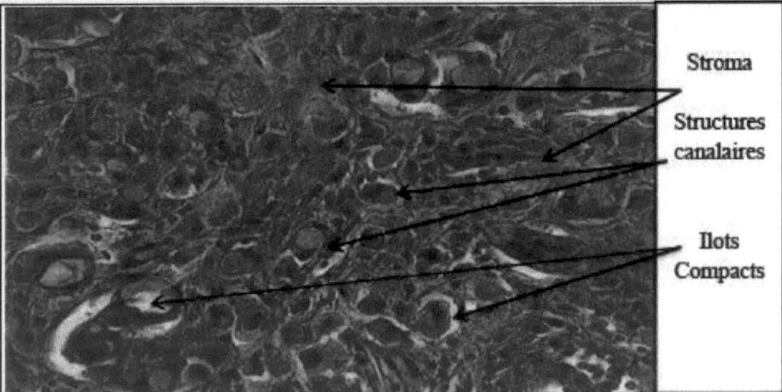

Figure 33: Histological section representing a grade II non-specific ductal carcinoma observed under the light microscope, stained with haematoxylin-eosin (Gr: 10×40) (Personal photo).

Invasive malignant epithelial cells form small ductal structures, compact islands and even dense sheets of cells. The stroma is often very fibrous.

Histopathological examination under the light microscope also enabled us to identify other histological types such as infiltrating lobular carcinoma. We will take as an example the patient (H2459) with a histopathological appearance of right breast infiltrating lobular carcinoma of Grade II according to SBR and PTNM stage (AJCC 8th edition 2017): T4N2aM1 (**Figure 34**).

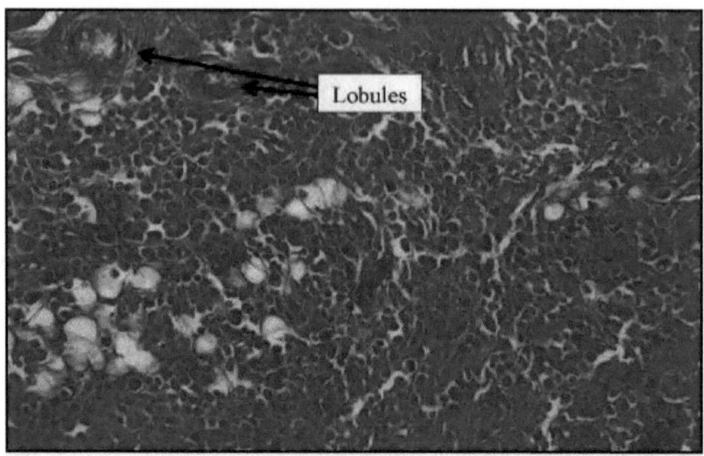

Figure 34: Histological section representing a grade II infiltrating lobular carcinoma observed under the light microscope, stained with haematoxylin-eosin (Gr: 10x40) (Personal photo).

VII.1.2 Results of the immunohistochemical study

Immunohistochemical examinations are necessary to determine the status of hormone and biological membrane receptor markers (HER2) and the restrogen and proliferation index (Ki67).

VII.1.2.1 HER2 status

Figure 35 shows the absence of membrane labelling, demonstrating incomplete weak expression of the HER2 antigen in <10% of tumour cells with a score of 0. Again for the same patient (H2459).

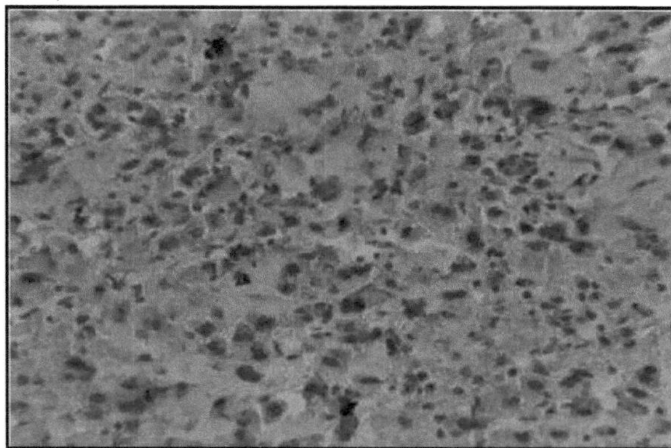

Figure 35: Invasive lobular carcinoma with HER2 iininiinostaining, Gr 40x10 (personal photo).

VII.1.2.2 Hormone receptors

Estrogen and progesterone receptors are detected in the nuclei of infiltrating tumour cells, and can also be detected in the surrounding normal breast tissue. This serves as an internal control.

We take the example of the patient (H2494) with a non-specific infiltrating ductal carcinoma with malignant proliferation of a highly infiltrative carcinomatous nature and atypical cells with enlarged irregular nuclei and appearance of a control on restrogen receptor immunostaining **(Figure 36).**

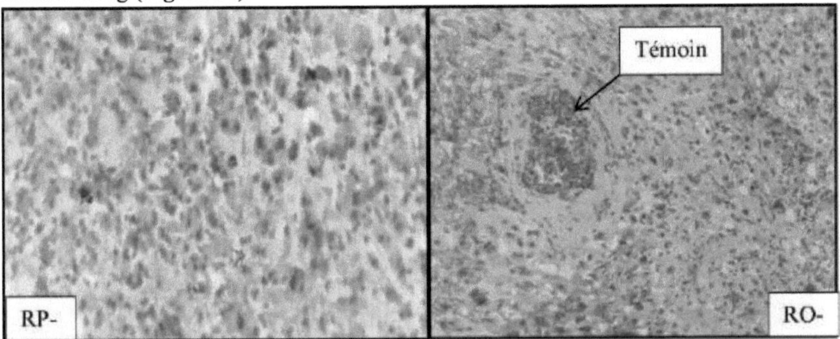

Figure 36: Nuclear immunolabelling of restrogen receptors in the presence of a control (right) and progesterone (left) 40 x10 (personal photo).

V II.2 Quantitative analysis results

V II.3.1 Descriptive study

V II.3.1.1 Trend in triple negatives from 2017-2022

The molecular classification of breast cancer has made it possible to divide the cases studied into the triple-negative breast cancer group (TNBC). According to the retrospective study we carried out for the last 6 years, we had an average of 47 for the year 2019 with a high rate of patients affected in the year 2021 with (22%), 2017 with (20%), 2022 with (15.3%) then 2018 with (10.2%), and finally (8.5%) for the year 2020 **(Table V). Table V: Trends in triple negatives from 2017-2022**

	Frequency	Percentage
Valid2017	12	20,3
2018	6	10,2
2019	14	23,7
2020	5	8,5
2021	13	22,0
2022	9	15,3
Total	59	100,0

This histogram shows a Gaussian curve, with the values distributed more or less symmetrically around the mean 47, with a standard deviation of 1.755 (**Figure 37**).

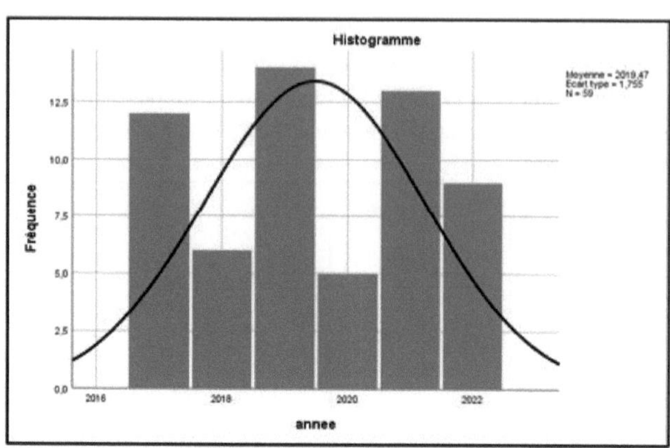

Figure 37: Trend in triple negatives from 2017-2022

VII.3.1.2 Age distribution of patients

We have a group of patients aged <50 years with a mean age of 42.36 years and a standard deviation of

of (5.495) means that the frequencies are dispersed **(Table VI).**

Table VI: Statistical distribution of patients by age.

Age		
N	Valid	59
M	oyenne	42,36
Median		42,00
Standard deviation		5,495

According to our study, patients in the 32-36 age group have the same frequencies (1.7%). The age group (38-39) also has fairly high frequencies of (11.9%) and (10.2%) respectively, and for people aged between 40 and 49 the frequencies vary between (3.4%) and (8.5%). These rates increase at the age of 50 with a frequency of (15.3%) **(Appendix VII), (Figure 38).**

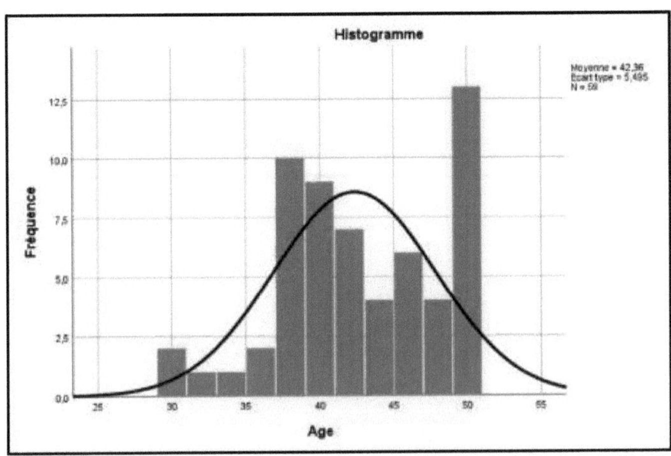

Figure 38: Age distribution of triple-negative breast cancer patients

VII.3.1.3 Breakdown of patients by sex

Breast cancer affects more women than men; in our study series, out of a total of 59 cases, 93.2% were women and 4 men accounted for the remaining 6.8% **(Table VII), (Figure 39).**

Table VII: Breakdown of patients by gender

	Frequency	Percentage
Valid Woman	55	93,2
Men	4	6,8
Total	59	100,0

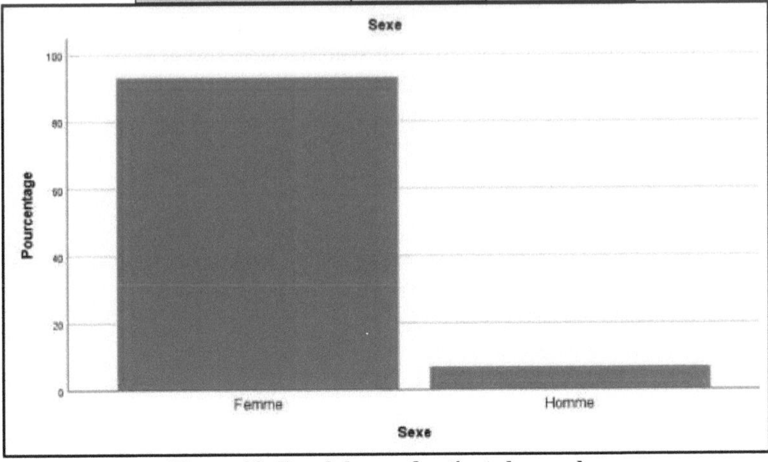

Figure 39: Breakdown of patients by gender

VII.3.1.4 Distribution of patients by tumour site

Based on the results of tumour positioning, we can say that the results were almost similar, with a frequency of (49.2%) of right tumour location for 29 cases and (50.8%) of left tumour location for 30 cases **(Table VIII), (Figure 40).**

Table VIII: Breakdown of patients by tumour site

	Frequency	Percentage
Valid Right	29	49,2
Left	30	50,8
Total	59	100,0

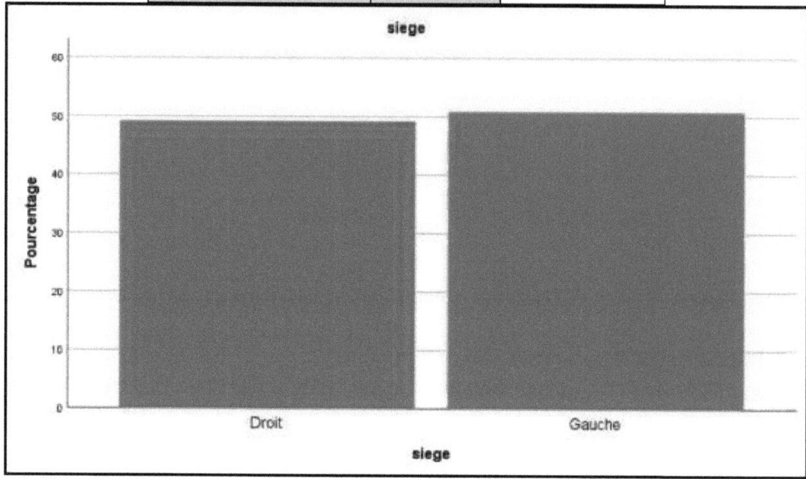

Figure 40: Distribution of patients by tumour site

VII.3.1.5 Distribution according to histological type

The majority of histological types of patients are infiltrating ductal carcinomas (IDC) (86.4%), while there is also a minority with a frequency of (10.2%) of histological type infiltrating lobular carcinomas (ILC).During our study we were able to count cases with both types with a frequency of (3.4%) **(Table IX), (Figure 41).**

Table IX: Breakdown of patients by histological type

		Frequency	Percentage
Valid	CCI	51	86,4
	CCI / CLI	2	3,4
	CLI	6	10,2
	Total	59	100,0

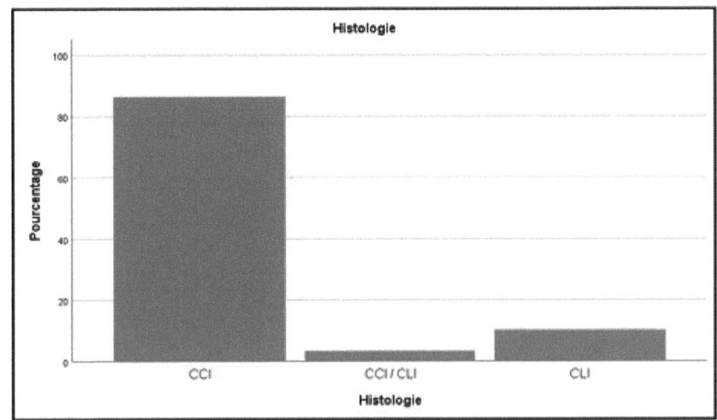

Figure 41: Distribution of patients with triple-negative breast cancer by histological type

VII.3.1.6 Breakdown by SBR grade

It was noted that the molecular sub-type of triple-negative breast cancer has a different SBR grade. Tumours belonging to this group were characterised by the intermediate histological grade SBR II (66.1% of cases), which represents the highest rate and is therefore the most frequent grade, in contrast to grade III (33.9% of cases) **(Table X)**, **(Figure 42).**

Table X: Breakdown of patients by SBR Grade

		Frequency	Percentage
Valid	II	39	66,1
	III	20	33,9
	Total	59	100,0

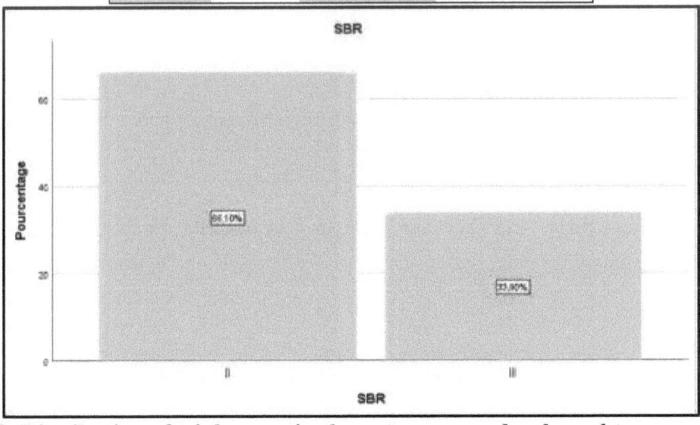

Figure 42: Distribution of triple-negative breast cancer molecular subtype as a function of SBR grade

VII.3.1.7 Distribution of patients according to tumour size

In this study, tumours classified as T2 predominated (66.1%), followed by tumours classified as T1 (25.4%), then tumours classified as T3 (5.1%), followed by tumours classified as T0 and T4 (1.7%) **(Table XI), (Figure 43).**

Table XI: Distribution of triple-negative breast cancers according to tumour size

		Frequency	Percentage
Valid	TO	1	1,7
	T1	15	25,4
	T2	39	66,1
	T3	3	5,1
	T4	1	1,7
	Total	59	100,0

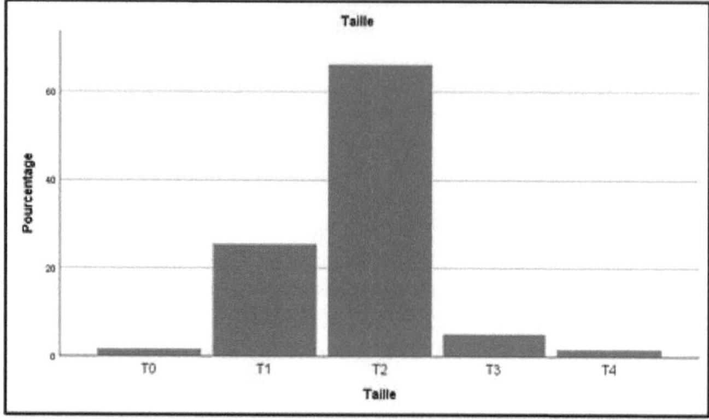

Figure 43: Distribution of patients by tumour size

VII.3.1.8 Distribution of patients according to lymph node involvement

Axillary lymph node metastases (EG+) were present in 88.1% of cases and absent (EG-) in 11.9% of patients (**Table XII**).

Table XII: Distribution of patients according to lymph node involvement

		Frequency	Percentage
Valid	EG+	52	88,1
	EG-	7	11,9
	Total	59	100,0

Axillary lymph node metastases (EG+) predominated in 52 of the 59 cases studied **(Figure 44).**

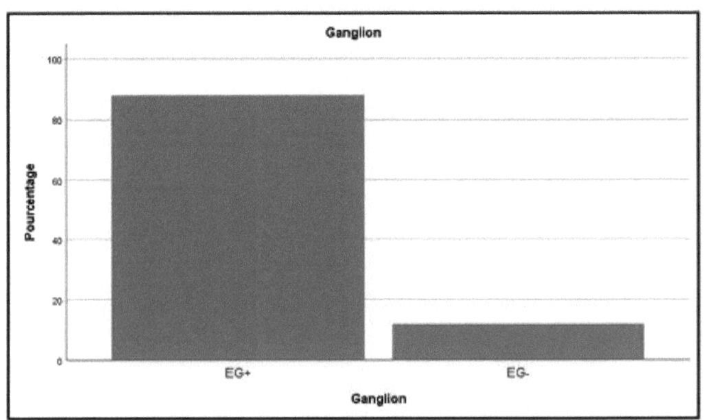

Figure 44: Distribution of patients according to lymph node involvement

VII.3.1.9 Distribution of patients according to distant metastases

Non-evaluable metastatic status (Mx) was present in 89.8% of patients followed by 10.2% of patients or metastatic status is present (M1) (**Table XIII**).

Table XIII: Distribution of patients according to distant metastases

		Frequency	Percentage
Valid	1	6	10,2
	x	53	89,8
	Total	59	100,0

Most metastases cannot be assessed (**Figure 45**).

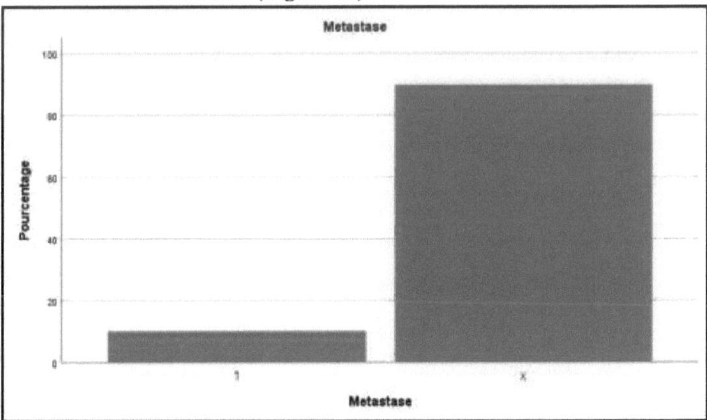

Figure 45: Distribution of patients according to distant metastases

VII.3.1.10 Breakdown of patients by type of surgery

Mastectomy involves removing the entire breast, unlike lumpectomy, which is therefore conservative surgery. Mastectomy has a higher frequency rate (89.8%), while lumpectomy is less frequent (10.2%) (**Table XIV**), **(Figure 46).**

Table XIV: Distribution of patients with triple-negative breast cancer by type of surgery

Surgery

		Frequency	Percentage
Valid	M	53	89,8
	T	6	10,2
	Total	59	100,0

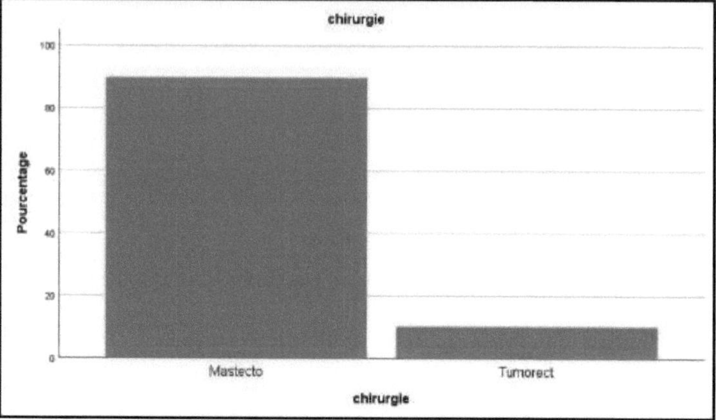

Figure 46: Distribution of patients according to surgical treatment

VII.3.2 Analytical study

VII.3.2.1 Distribution of tumours by histological type according to age

Estimation of the number of patients as a function of age clearly shows the dispersion of histological types in the different patients in the three groups. **Table XV** shows this variability within the young patients < 50 years of age. However, this relationship is quite strong, as shown by a cramer V (0.502) and Phi(0.710), which is a measure derived from the X^2 , with a significance level of $p<0.05$ we can deduce that there is a significant difference **(Appendix V), (Table XV).**

Table XV: Table of symmetrical measures of tumour distribution by histological type according to age

Symmetrical measurements			
		Value	Approximate meaning
Nominal per Nominal	Phi	0,710	0,759
	V de Cramer	0,502	0,759
N of valid observations		59	

The results show that the infiltrating ductal carcinoma (IDC) histological type is the most important, especially for patients aged 38 and 50, followed by the infiltrating lobular carcinoma (ILCC) histological type for a group of patients aged 35, 37, 42, 43, 49 and 50, and for the groups with both histological types, most are aged 39 or 45 (**Figure 47**).

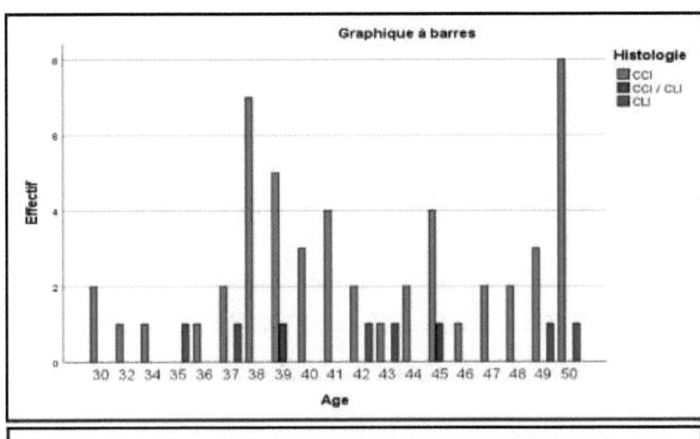

Figure 47 : Répartition des tumeurs selon le type histologique en fonction d'âge

VII.3.2.2 Distribution of tumours by histological type and sex

Our study shows that all male patients with triple-negative breast cancer have the histological type invasive ductal carcinoma (IDC), both male and female patients 47 have invasive ductal carcinoma and 6 patients have invasive lobular carcinoma (ILC) as well as both histological types (**Table XVI**).

Table XVI: Distribution of tumours by histological type and sex

Workforce				
		Gender		Total
		Woman	Men	
Histology	CCI	47	4	51
	CCI / CLI	2	0	2
	CLI	6	0	6
Total		55	4	59

In this case, the statistical value (χ^2 =0.673) is lower than the threshold value (χ^2 =3.84) with a ddl= 2, so we can say that there is no significant difference, (**Table XVII**).

Table XVII: Chi-square tests for the distribution of tumours by histological type according to sex

Chi-square tests			
	Value	ddl	Asymptotic significance (bilateral)
Pearson chi-square	0,673[a]	2	0,714
Likelihood ratio	1,210	2	0,546
N of valid observations	59		
A 4 cells (66.7%) have a theoretical size of less than 5. The minimum theoretical number of cells is 0.14.			

On this table of symmetrical measures we have the same phi and V values of carmer, which means that there is a weak relationship between the variables, bearing in mind that the headcount for women with infiltrating ductal carcinomas is much higher than for men **(Figure 48), (Table XVIII)**.

Table XVIII Table of symmetrical measures of tumour distribution by histological type according to sex

Symmetrical measurements			
		Value	Approximate meaning
Nominal per Nominal	Phi	0,107	0,714
	V de Cramer	0,107	0,714
N of valid observations		59	

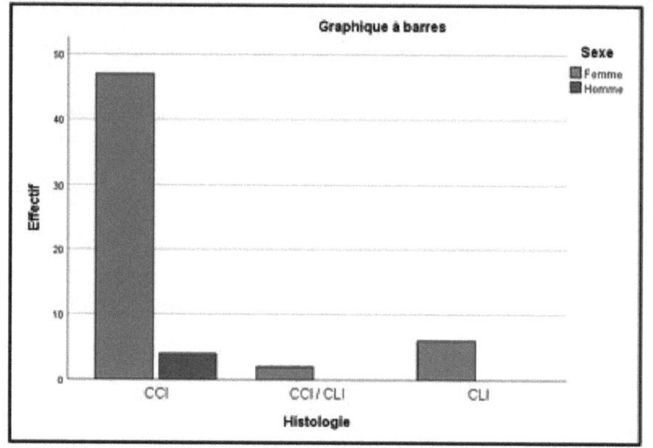

Figure 48: Distribution of tumours by histological type and sex

VII.3.2.3 Distribution of triple-negative breast cancer tumours according to tumour site

If we classify the tumours according to tumour site, we first have infiltrating ductal carcinomas, which are the most frequent histological type to be found in both the left and right breast, with the vast majority in the left tumour site, while the small number of infiltrating lobular carcinomas (ILC) are equally divided between the right and left sites **(Table XIX)**.

Table XIX: Distribution of tumours according to tumour site

Histology * Siege cross-tabulation				
Workforce				
		Seat		Total
		Law	Left	
Histology	CCI	24	27	51
	CCI / CCL	2	0	2
	CCL	3	3	6
Total		29	30	59

The Phi and V values of cramer are identical with (0.19), so we can say that there is a weak relationship between the variables, so there is no significant difference. This explains why the tumours are not necessarily located at the same tumour site **(Table XX), (Figure 49). Table XX: Symmetrical measures of tumour distribution according to tumour site**

Symmetrical measurements			
		Value	Approximate meaning
Nominal per Nominal	Phi	0,191	0,340
	V de Cramer	0,191	0,340
N of valid observations		59	

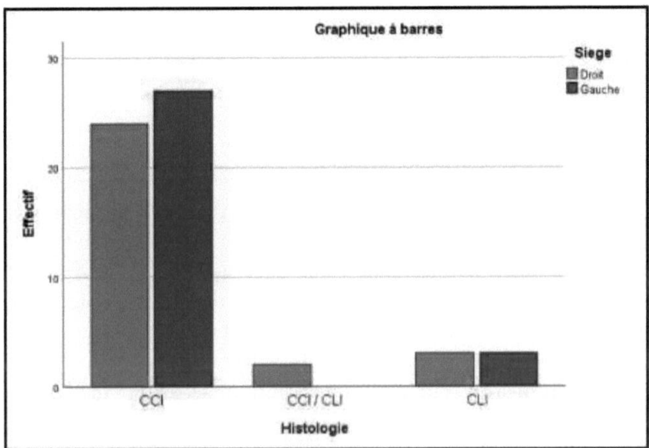

Figure 49: Distribution of tumours by tumour site

VII.3.2.4 Distribution of tumours according to SBR stage

With a total of 51 patients with infiltrating ductal carcinomas (IDC), the majority of patients are SBR II (35 patients) and the remaining 16 patients are SBR III, in contrast to patients with infiltrating lobular carcinomas, 2 patients are stage II and 4 patients are stage III (**Table XXI**),(**Figure 50**).

Table XXI: Breakdown of patients by SBR stage

Histology * SBR cross-tabulation

Workforce

		SBR		Total
		II	III	
Histology	CCI	35	16	51
	CCI / CLI	2	0	2
	CLI	2	4	6
Total		39	20	59

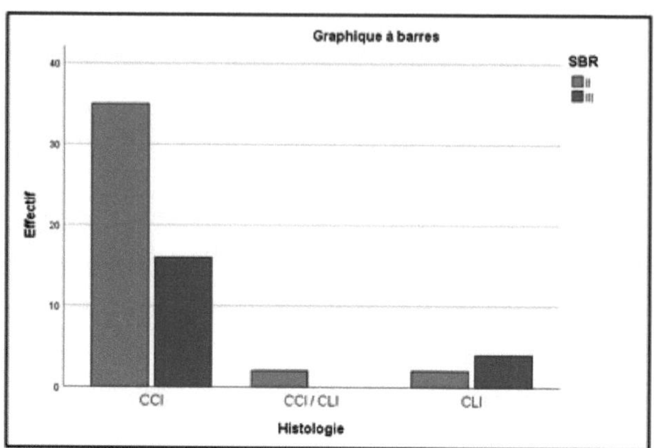

Figure 50: Distribution of triple-negative breast cancer patients according to SBR stage

According to the table below, we have the value of X^2 (4.046), so it is greater than 3.841, which is the threshold degree with a ddl= 2, which means that there is a significant difference, not forgetting that the Phi and the carmer value are equal (0.262), so we can deduce that the correlation between the variables is average (**Table XXII**).

Table XXII: Statistical measures of patient distribution according to SBR Grade

Chi-square tests				
		Value	ddl	Asymptotic significance (bilateral)
Pearson chi-square		4,046[a]	2	,132
Likelihood ratio		4,475	2	,107
N of valid observations		59		
a. 4 cells (66.7%) have an ef		Theoretical headcount less than 5. The minimum theoretical number of employees is .68.		
Symmetrical measurements				
			Value	Approximate meaning
Nominal per Nominal	Phi		0,262	,132
	V de Cramer		0,262	,132
N of valid observations			59	

VII.3.2.5 Distribution of tumours according to histological type and tumour size

T2 tumour size is the most dominant in patients with invasive ductal carcinoma, followed by T1 tumour size, 14 of whom have the same histological type (ICC).14 In patients with invasive lobular carcinoma, the majority have a T2 tumour size **(Table XXIII)**.

Table XXIII: Distribution of tumours according to tumour size

Histology crosstab * Size							
Workforce							
		Size					Total
		T0	T1	T2	T3	T4	
Histology	CCI	1	14	33	3	0	51

	CCI / CLI	0	0	2	0	0	2
	CLI	0	1	4	0	1	6
Total		1	15	39	3	1	59

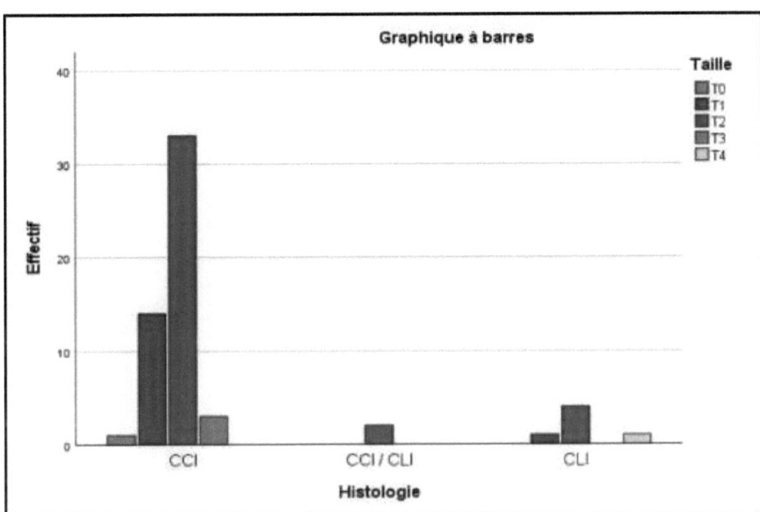

Figure 51: Distribution of tumours by histological type and tumour size

We have an $X^2 = 10.596$, with a ddl of 8, so there is a significant difference between histological type and tumour size (**Table XXIV**).

Table XXIV: Chi-square test for the distribution of patients according to tumour size

Chi-square tests			
	Value	ddl	Asymptotic significance (bilateral)
Pearson chi-square	10,596[a]	8	,226
Likelihood ratio	7,356	8	,499
N of valid observations	59		
a. 13 cells (86.7%) have a theoretical number less than 5. The minimum theoretical number of cells is .03.			

VII.3.2.6 Distribution of tumours according to histological type and lymph node involvement

In our series of studies, 52 patients with invasive ductal carcinoma (IDC) had lymph node involvement.

Table XXV: Distribution of patients according to histological type and lymph node involvement

Histology cross-tabulation * Ganglion
Workforce

		Ganglion		Total
		EG+	EG-	
Histology	CCI	44	7	51
	CCI / CLI	2	0	2
	CLI	6	0	6
Total		52	7	59

The statistical value (X^2 =1.246) is lower than the threshold value (X^2 =3.84). We conclude that there is no significant difference between histological type and lymph node involvement of the tumour (**Table XXVI**),(**Figure 52**).

Table XXVI: Distribution of patients by histological type according to lymph node involvement, using chi-square test

Chi-square tests			
	Value	ddl	Asymptotic significance (bilateral)
Pearson chi-square	1,246[a]	2	,536
Likelihood ratio	2,183	2	,336
N of valid observations	59		
a. 3 cells (50.0%) have a theoretical size of less than 5. The minimum theoretical number of cells is .24.			

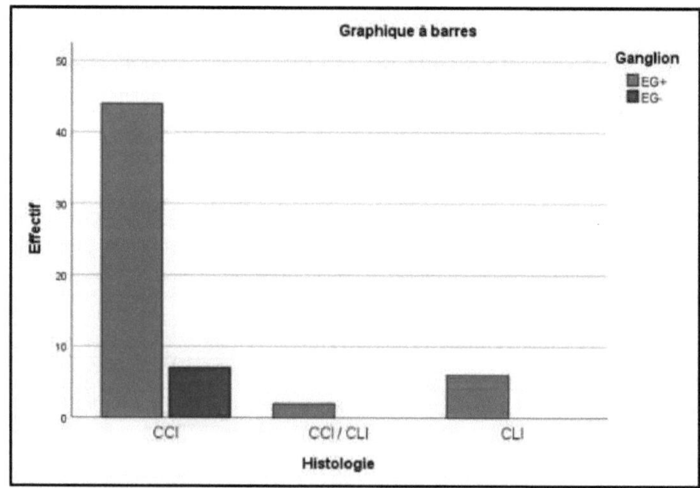

Figure 52: Distribution of patients according to lymph node involvement

VII.3.2.7 Distribution of tumours by histological type according to metastatic status

Histological type as a function of metastatic status did not represent any significant difference, which can be explained by the statistical value of (X^2 = 11.672), ddl=2 and risk of error 5% **(Table XXVII).**

Table XXVII: Chi-square test for the distribution of patients according to metastatic status

Chi-square tests

	Value	ddl	Asymptotic significance (bilateral)
Pearson chi-square	11,672[a]	2	0,003
Likelihood ratio	7,660	2	0,022
N of valid observations	59		
a. 3 cells (50.0%) have a theoretical size of less than 5. The number of cells is .20.			minimum theoretical f

The correlation statistics showed that the two values of Phi and V of carmer are identical, which means that there is a dependency **(Table XXVIII)**.

Table XXVIII: Symmetrical measure of distribution of patients with triple-negative breast cancer according to metastatic status

Symmetrical measurements			
		Value	Approximate meaning
Nominal per Nominal	Phi	,445	,003
	V de Cramer	,445	,003
N of valid observations		59	

In conclusion, the metastasis status of the patients studied could not be assessed for most patients with infiltrating ductal carcinomas, unlike infiltrating lobular carcinomas, with a fairly low number of patients for both Mx and M1 (presence of metastases).
(Figure 53).

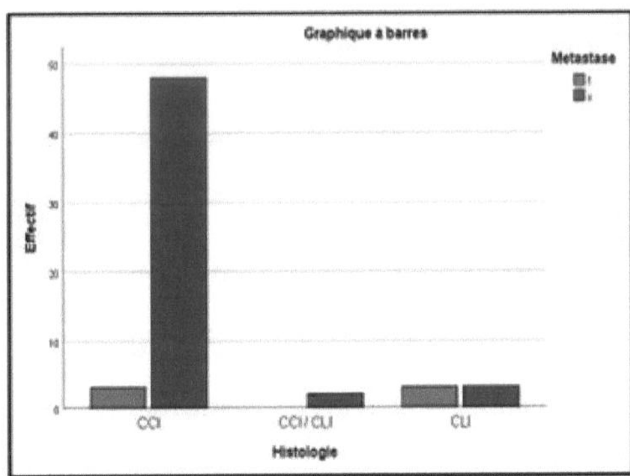

Figure 53: Distribution of triple-negative breast cancer patients according to metastatic status

VII.3.2.8 Distribution of patients according to surgical treatment

The most frequent surgical treatment is mastectomy, and after performing a chi-square test we can say that there is a significant difference with a value of X^2 =1.048 which is lower than the X^2 threshold with a ddl =2 and a risk of error of 5% **(Table XXIX), (Figure 54).**

Table XXIX: Chi-square test used to study the distribution of patients according to surgical treatment

	Value	ddl	Asymptotic significance

			(bilateral)
Pearson chi-square	1,048[a]	2	,592
Likelihood ratio	1,852	2	,396
N of valid observations	59		
a. 3 cells (50.0%) have a theoretical size of less than 5. The minimum theoretical number of cells is .20.			

The results of the two values are identical with a value of Phi and V of carmer (0.133), so we can say that there is a low correlation between the variables (**Table XXX**).

Table XXX: Symmetrical measurements of patient distribution according to surgical treatment

Symmetrical measurements			
		Value	Approximate meaning
Nominal per Nominal	Phi	0,133	,592
	V de Cramer	0,133	,592
N of valid observations		59	
c. Correlation statistics are only available for numerical data.			

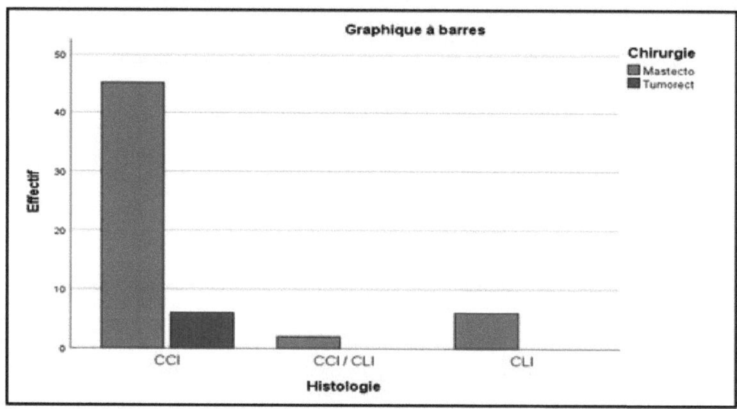

Figure 54: Distribution of patients according to surgical treatment

CHAPTER VIII

DISCUSSION

Over the last 6 years, the evolution of breast cancer pathology has been analysed to identify prognostic factors, while defining an adapted and targeted treatment to reduce the severity of the disease. Our study was carried out on a population in western Algeria comprising 59 patients with triple-negative breast cancer aged < 50 years.

In our present study we found a percentage of 6.8% of male patients, this frequency is inconsistent with the literature. Charu and colleagues noted that triple-negative breast cancer may be more common in young men with breast cancer with a percentage of 26% in a population of 500 patients per year, so this means that there is a discrepancy **(Charu A et *al.* , 2021).**

The frequency of breast cancer in young women varies according to researchers. In France, it is estimated at 10% according to **(Molinié ,2019)**.according to Anders, 6.6% in the United States(USA) **(Anders C et *al.* , 2009)**.in our series, this frequency was 93.2% for triple-negative breast cancers in a population of 59 cases. This difference in frequency could be identified by the difference in age pyramids between the populations.

The study we carried out showed a frequency of 3.4% and 8.5% for the 40-49 age group, but in a study carried out by other researchers, they noted that the 40-49 age group was affected in a comparable way (24 versus 29%). Thus, women aged between 40 and 59, representing 53% of our population, are at higher risk of TNBC. In addition, 15 patients (17%) were under 40 years of age **(Darouich S et *al.* , 2017).**

Our total sample is 59 patients, of which the percentage is of the order of 86.4% (51 cases), grades II and III present 66.1% and 33.5%.Comparing with the study of **(Belouad M , 2018)** infiltrating ductal carcinoma is the most predominant type represents 68.3% of cases with a mean tumour size of 30 mm. Histopronostic grades II and III account for 43.2% and 56.8% of cases respectively. According to the literature, women aged 35 and under have a significantly higher rate of lobular carcinomas (7.5%), compared with 10.2% in our study series. **(Chan A et al. , 2000).**

In our series, the tumours were classified as T2 (66.1%), followed by T1 (25.4%) and T3 (5.1%). Only T0 and T4 tumours were present (1.7%).

Other studies have been done by researchers **(Darouich S et al. , 2017)** who had noted that the mean clinical tumour size was 3.63 cm (1.5-15 cm) and the majority T2 tumour status with (41%), which agrees with our results.

In the light of our results, we found 88.1% of our 52 patients to have lymph node involvement compared with 44% in the study by Foulkes et al. The relationship between triple-negative breast cancer (TNBC) and lymph node metastases is less clearly established; lymph node status does not seem to correlate with tumour size **(Foulkes W et *al.*, 2003).**

In our present study, the metastatic status was 89.9% of non-evaluable metastases and 10.2% of patients had M1 metastases. In contrast, a Moroccan study showed that the diagnosis of breast cancer was early in 56.9% of cases, compared with 43.1% which were late. 51.6% of patients had lymph node involvement and 7.7% developed distant metastases **(Ahmadaye I, et *al.* , 2016).**

In our retrospective study, mastectomy was more frequent (89.8%), whereas lumpectomy was less frequent (10.2%). In the study by Darouich and colleagues, lumpectomy was performed after neoadjuvant chemotherapy in two patients and followed by mastectomy after adjuvant

chemotherapy in two other patients. A Patey-type radical mastectomy was performed in 44 patients (54%), post neoadjuvant chemotherapy in 15 patients, including two in palliative situation **(Darouich S et *al.* , 2017)**.
In 2017, a study was conducted in 468 patients with advanced triple-negative breast cancer who had already received several lines of treatment **(Champion E , 2021).**
Despite advances in treatment and the emergence of targeted therapies, breast cancer remains the leading cause of death in women **(Belouad M , 2018).**
In Algeria, according to Algerian oncologists and surgeons, most patients diagnosed with triple-negative breast cancer are considered to be in a serious and very advanced state, and treatment is based on chemotherapy. Platinum-based treatment is recommended in cases of proven BRCA mutation **(Bendib A et al. , 2016).** Among other things, this is a particularly difficult form of the disease to treat, paradoxically transforming the mutation of this gene into a 'protective' factor, and above all it is particularly difficult to decide to apply a preventive treatment to a healthy population **(Zitouni M et *al.* , 2017).**

CHAPTER IX

CONCLUSION & OUTLOOK

Triple-negative tumours represent a subgroup of breast cancers associated with a poor prognosis. They are defined immunohistochemically by the absence of restrogen, progesterone and HER2 receptor expression. Given the non-response of TNBCs to hormone therapy, chemotherapy remains the only systemic treatment for these tumours.

Analysis of the results of our present study and the data in the literature show that triple-negative breast cancer is characterised by greater clinical aggressiveness and a poor prognosis despite the use of chemotherapy. While this subtype frequently responds to neoadjuvant chemotherapy, the prognosis for these patients remains poor, and there is a need for more aggressive strategies and the development of molecular signatures associated with targeted therapies.

Such an approach cannot be achieved without optimal biological characterisation, enabling the complexity of this sub-group of tumours to be understood. This requires the collaboration of a multidisciplinary team in clinical trials involving anatomopathologists, oncologists and basic researchers.

Triple-negative breast cancer is currently the subject of several clinical trials, which are listed in a national register accessible to the public.

BIBLIOGRAPHICAL REFERENCES

Abid L, (Department of Visceral Surgery, Hôpital Bologhine), No. 16060 (March 2002).

Ahmadaye I, Bendahhou K, Mstaghanmi H, Saile R, and Benider A. "Breast cancer in Morocco: phenotypic profile of tumors." , 2016.

Anders C, Johnson R, Litton J, Phillips M, Bleyer A, "Breast Cancer Before Age 40 years Seminars in Oncology. , 2009: 237 - 249.

Azam S , Lange T, Huynh S, Aro A.R, von Euler-Chelpin M, Vejborg I, Tj0nneland A, Lynge E, and Andersen, Z.J. "Hormone replacement therapy mammohgraohic density and breast cancer risk a cohort study cancer causes control." 29(6), n° 10.1007 (, 2018): 495-505.

Barouagui S., Zaoui C ,Senhadji R ,El Kébir F.Z ,Koudjeti R. "Overweight and breast cancer in western Algeria." *35° Journées de la Société Française de Sénologie et de Pathologie Mammaire*, , 2013.

Belouad M. "Triple-negative breast cancer, experience of the MED V Rabat military hospital: about 52 cases." , 2018.

Bendib A., Sami S, Admane S, Afiane Z,Amani A,Bendib A. "Manual de Prise en Charge." , 2016.

Boughera N,. "CHUC." 2012.

Boulton SJ. "BRCA1-Mediated Ubiquitylation Cell cycle. , 2006.

Brux J, and Hollmann K.H. *Histopathology of the breast.* 1979.

Champion E. "TRIPLE NEGATIVE BREAST CANCER: AN EFFECTIVE THERAPEUTIC INNOVATION CHANGES THE GAME". , 2021.

Chan A ,Xiaolong Wang, Tong Chen, Wenhao Li, Qifeng yang. "Breast cancer in woman aged 35 years and less." *a single institution*, , 2000.

Charu A, Shah N, Markham J, Rodriguez C,. oncologist video coference on triple negative breast cancer in men , 2021.

Chen CF , Li S Y, Chen PL, Chen ZD, Sharp WH, Lee. "The nuclear localization sequences of the BRCA1 protein interact with the importin-alpha subnit of the nuclear transport signal receptor." *J Biol Chem*, , 1996: 32863-32868.

Cherbal F, Salhi N,Houamel DAE, Chikh A,Guettouche S,Belomokhtar S,Chibane A,Bakour E,Benhassina T,Toulas C,Boualgua K,Cherifi A. "BRCA1 and BRCA2 mutations bresat cancer report of screeing." , 2015.

Chéreau E. "specificity of breast cancer management in young women." *Hôpital Saint Joseph Marseille*, May ,2019.

Darouich S , Olfa elAmine E, Betaieb I, Dhiab T, Rahal K, Gamoudi A. "triple-negative breast cancer: clinical-epidemiological study and." *LA TUNISIE MEDICALE*, , 2017.

Esashi F , Chris N, J Gannon Y,Liu T, Hunt M, Jain SC, West. "Dependent phosphorylation of BRCA2 as a regulatory mechanism for recombinational repair." *Nature*, , 2005: 598-604.

Fackenthal J and Olopade I,Breast cancer risk associated with BRCA1 and BRCA2 in diverse populations , 2007.

Foulkes W , Matcalfe K, W Hanna, HT Lunch, P Ghadirian, N Tung. "Disruption of the expected positive correlation between breast tumor size and lymph node status in BRCA-1 related breast carcinoma." , 2003.

Franchet C , Duprez-Paumier R,Lacroix-Triki M. "Molecular taxonomy of luminal breast cancer." (Bull Cancer 2015) , 2015: 34-46.

Freres P , Collignon J,Gennigens C, Scagnol I,Rorive A,Barbeaux A,Coucke P.A,Jérusalem

G. "Le cancer du sein triple négatif. , 2010: 120-126.

Goldhirsch A, Wood WC,Coates AS, Gelber RD, Thurlimann B, Senn HJ, Panel MSrategies. "Gallen international expret consensus on the primary therapy of Early Breast Cancer." 22 (, 2011): 1736-1747.

Hamajima N , Hirose, K., Tajima, K., Rohan, T., Calle, E.E., Heath, C.W., Coates, R.J., Liff,. "and Collaborative Group on Hormonal Factors ,Alcohol, tobacco and breast cancer." *IARC working Group on the Evaluation of Carcinogenic Risk to humans*, No. 10.1038/sj.bjc.6600596 (,2002): 1234-1245.

Henderson. ,2012.

Kelsey JL;Bernstein L,. "Epidemiology and prevention of breast cancer." *Ann Rev PubL health*, 1996: 47-67.

Key TJ , Verkasalo PK, Banks E. "Banks E.Epidemiology of breast." *Cancer Lancet Oncol*, , 2001: 133-40.

Lacroixi, M, and F Penault. "TNM classification for breast cancer 8th edition." , 2017.

Lee LH , Yang H,Bigras G. "Current breast cancer proliferative markers correlate variably based on descoupled duration of cell cycle phases." *Sci Rep*, , 2014.

Liedtke C , Mazouni C, Hess KR, André F, Tordai A, Mejia JA, Syammns WF, Gonzalez-Angulo AM. "Response to neoadjuvant therapy and long-term survival in patients with triplenegative breast cancer." 8 (, 2008): 1275-81.

Mokrane F. "Breast cancer. ,2020.

Nai'bo P,. "triple negative breast cancer natural history and study of genetic factors involved." *life sciences*, 2018.

Péro , "Molecular portraits of natural human mammary tumours." 2000: 474-752.

Pinder SE , Paish CE,Bell J, Blamey R,Robertson JF , Nicholason RI,Ellis IO. "Expression of luminal and basal cytokenatins in hummain breast carcinoma." *J Pathol*, , 2004: 661-671.

Prat , 2010,Lehmann et al,2011,Chen et al,2012,Prat et al,2013,Lehmann et al,2015. , 2010.

Reis F , Tutt,Nishimura,Arima,Cheang,Rakha ,Foulkes,Characteristics of triple-negative breast cancer, 2011.

Rochefort H , Jacques Rouëssé, M R.M. Ancelle-Park, C. Hill, H. Sancho-Garnier, D. Stoppa-Lyonnet, A. Tardivon, D. Birnbaum, Ph. Bouchard, J. Estève, Ph. Jeanteur, Y. Le Bouc, H. Léridon, T. Maudelonde, G. Schaison, M. Tubiana. "Breast cancer incidence and prevention" *bullet from the French National Academy of Medicine*, 2008.

Villarreal C , Aguila C, Magallanes MC,Mohar A, Bargallo E, Meneses A,. "Breast cancer in young women in latin America." *groming burgen oncologist*, , 2013.

Wooster R , Neuhausen SL, Quirk Y, GM Lenoir, Lynch H, Feunteun J, Devillee P, Cornelisse CJ, Menko FH, Daly PA, Ormiston W, McManus R, Pye C, Lewis CM, Cannon-Albright L, Peto J,Ponder BAJ, Skolnick MH, Easton DF, Goldgar DE,Stratton MR, R Wooster, SL Neuhausen,J Mangion, Y Quirk. "Localization of a breast cancer susceptibility gene BRCA2 to chromosome 13q12-13." *Science*, , 1994.

Zafrani B, Mac GroGan Gaetan , Salomon Anne Vincent ,Arnould Laurant. *Enseingement Post-Universitaire de Pathologie Mammaire.* Bordaux , Paris: International Academy of Pathology, ,2007.

Zitouni M , Grangaud J,Cherf-Bouzida F. "Epidemiological data on cancer in eastern and south-eastern Algeria." , 2017.

INTERNET SITES

[1] : http://www.depistagesein.ca/anatomie-du-sein/#.YmFM1ipzzIU

[2] :https://www.informationhospitaliere.com/le-cancer-du-sein-depistage-et-traitement-de-la- illness

[3] :https://www.docteur-eric-sebban.fr/cancer-du-sein/diagnostic-cancer-sein/anatomie-et-pathologies-du-sein/

[4] :https://cancer.ca/fr/cancer-information/cancer-types/breast/what-is-breast-cancer/cancerous-tumours/ductal-carcinoma

[5]:https://rubanrose.org/blogue/cancer-du-sein-inflammatoire-un-cancer-rare-et-agressif/

[6] :https://cancer.ca/fr/cancer-information/cancer-types/breast/what-is-breast-cancer/cancerous-tumours/paget-disease-of-the-breast

[7] : https://www.sciencedirect.com/science/article/pii/S1631069106001910

[8] : http://www.ligue-cancer21.info/actualites/comment-une-cellule-devient-elle-cancereuse/

[9] : https://www.who.int/fr/news-room/fact-sheets/detail/breast-cancer

[10] :https://gco.iarc.fr/today/data/factsheets/cancers/20-Breast-fact-sheet.pdf?fbclid=IwAR1dcsXV5xIU0KzrFTSmsHBWQ0qAhPlN_D3Hw7aP08sjgxMcZic7RQSDisI

[11] :https://www.aps.dz/sante-science-technologie/128390-cancer-en-algerie-65-000-new-cases-since-begin-2021

[12] https://www.panafrican-med-journal.com/content/article/38/88/full/

[13] :http://www.dknews-dz.com/article/131133-cancer-du-sein-plus-de-400-nouveaux-cas-en-2020-a-oran.html

[14] :https://www.gyneco-online.com/cancerologie/specificite-de-la-prise-en-charge-du-cancer-du-sein-chez-la-femme-jeune

[15] :https://cancerdusein.predilife.com/lincidence-de-lage-en-matiere-de-cancer-du-sein/

[16] :https://cancer.ca/fr/cancer-information/cancer-types/breast/what-is-breast-cancer/breast-cancer-in-men

[17] :https://cancer.ca/fr/cancer-information/what-is-cancer/genes-and-cancer/genetic-changes-and-cancer-risk

[18] :https://www.e-cancer.fr/Patients-et-proches/Les-cancers/Cancer-du-sein/Facteurs-de-risk/Genetic predispositions

[19] :http://www.depistagesein.ca/risques-familiaux/#.Yn694CpzzIU

[20] :https://www.euro.who.int/fr/media-centre/sections/press-releases/2021/alcohol-is-one-of-the-biggest-risk-factors-for-breast-cancer

[21] : https://www.nicorette.fr/je-songe-a-m-arreter/les-effets-de-l-arret/menopause-et-tabac

[22] : https://www.cancer-environnement.fr/144-cancer-du-sein.ce.aspx

[23] :https://www.bioalaune.com/fr/actualite-bio/11969/17-substances-chimiques-qui-promote-brinch-cancer

[24] :https://www.clubic.com/sante/article-886696-1-ondes-electromagnetiques-comment-reduce-exposure.html

[25] : https://www.cancer-environnement.fr/604-Champs-electromagnetiques.ce.aspx

[26] : https://www.ipubli.inserm.fr/bitstream/handle/10608/5450/MS_2005_2_175.html

[27] : https://sante.journaldesfemmes.fr/fiches-sexo-gyneco

[28] https://cancer.ca/fr/cancer-information/cancer-types/breast/staging

[29] : https://cancer.ca/fr/treatments/tests-and-procedures/hormone-receptor-status-test
[30] : https://www.fondation-arc.org/traitements-soins-cancer/hormonotherapie/quest-ce-que-hormone therapy
[31] :http://www.depistagesein.ca/types-de-cancer-du-sein/#.YmNEfCpzzIU
[32] : https://ishh.fr/cancer-du-sein/le-cancer-du-sein-lobulaire/
[33] : http://www.depistagesein.ca/carcinome-infiltrant/#.YoAPHypzzIU
[34] : http://www.depistagesein.ca/carcinome-infiltrant/#.YmNKhypzzIU
[35] :https://cancer.ca/fr/cancer-information/cancer-types/breast/what-is-breast-cancer/cancerous-tumours/paget-disease-of-the-breast
[36] : https://www.edimark.fr/Front/frontpost/getfiles/25293.pdf
[37] :https://www.roche.fr/fr/patients/info-patients-cancer/diagnostic-cancer/diagnostic-breast-cancer/her2.html
[38] :https://www.roche.fr/fr/patients/info-patients-cancer/diagnostic-cancer/diagnostic-breast-cancer/her2.html
[39] :https://www.edimark.fr/Front/frontpost/getfiles/25292.pdf
[40] : https://curie.fr/dossier-pedagogique/pas-un-mais-des-cancers-du-sein
[41] :https://www.roche.fr/fr/patients/info-patients-cancer/comprendre-cancer/cancer-du-sein-triple-negatives.html
[42] :https://tel.archives-ouvertes.fr/tel-01561011/file/2016_TOLZA_archivage.pdf
[43] :https://pubmed.ncbi.nlm.nih.gov/21633166/
[44] : https://www.nature.com/articles/nrc2054
[45] :https://www.researchgate.net/figure/BRCA1-and-BRCA2-functional-domains-a-The-BRCA1-amino-terminus-contains-a-RING-domain_fig2_224824106
[46] : https://medicalforum.ch/fr/detail/doi/fms.2017.03056
[47] : https://www.cancer.be/le-cancer/metastase
[48] : https://www.arcagy.org/infocancer/localisations/cancers-feminins/cancer-du-sein
[49] :https://www.santelog.com/actualites/cancer-du-sein-une-nano-therapie-contre-les-tumour-aggression
[50] :https://ishh.fr/cancer-du-sein/les-therapies-ciblees-dans-le-traitement-du-cancer-du-sein/
[51] :https://www.chudequebec.ca/getmedia/e7486d22-9e68-48ee-a1e9-a9453aeb9070/8h45-dre-anne-choquette-presentation-er-pr-et-her2.aspx
[52] :https://acthera.univ-lille.fr/co/Bevacizumab__AVASTINJ__1.html
[53] :https://www.roche.fr/fr/patients/info-patients-cancer/comprendre-cancer/cancer-du-sein-triple-negatives.html
[54] https://www.cancertreatmentreviews.com/article/S0305-7372(15)00151-6/fulltext
[55] :https://docplayer.fr/44268035-Traitements-systemiques-dans-le-cancer-du-sein-actualites-lionel-duck-et-renaud-poncin-oncologues-clinique-saint-pierre-ottignies-26-may-2016.html
[56] : https://www.anticorps-enligne.fr/resources/17/1216/immunohistochimie-ihc/

Annex I

Questionnaire cancer:

Nom prénom (initiales): fait à Oran le/ /

Date et lieu de naissance: **sexe:** F M

Etat civil: **Année de mariage:**

Age des premières règles: **Poids:** **Taille:**

Nombre de grossesses: **Année de 1ère G** **NFC:** **ND:**

Prise de contraceptifs oraux (marque): oui non

Ménopause: oui non

Age:

Prise de THS (marque): oui non

Groupe sanguin: A B AB O + –

Antécédents familiaux (cancers dans la famille) oui non

Type: **organes atteints:** **quel parent atteint?**

Niveau économique: **activité professionnelle:**

Sein atteint: Droit Gauche Les deux

Taille de la tumeur:

Existence de métastases: Oui Non

Organes touchés

Autre pathologie diagnostiquées:

Paramètres anatomopathologiques

Année de la découverte du cancer et type de cancer diagnostiqué:

Grade du cancer: I II III

Histologie:

Annex II

Table XXXI: Stages of breast cancer (Zafrani B et *al.* ,2007).

Stadiums	Locations
Stage 0 (Cancer in situ)	Tumour remains localised in the canal where it originated. The tumour is non-invasive and has not spread beyond the basement membrane (Tis NO M0).
Stage I (Tumour measures 2 cm or less)	Tumour < 2 cm, no palpable lymph nodes, no distant metastases (T1 N0 M0).
Stage II (2 types of tumour)	Tumour < 5 cm with invasion of 1 to 3 axillary lymph nodes or involvement of the internal mammary sentinel lymph nodes (mobile axillary), without metastases (T0/1/2 N1 M0);or tumour > 2 cm, without lymph node involvement, without metastases (T2/3 N0 M0)
Stage III	Any tumour, without metastases, with : -At least 4 axillary nodes affected or clinical internal mammary invasion or involvement of sub-clavicular lymph nodes or homolateral supra-clavicular lymph nodes (all T N2/3 M0) or tumour with direct extension to the chest wall or skin or inflammatory tumour (T4 all N M0) or tumour > 5 cm with invasion of 1 to 3 axillary lymph nodes or involvement of internal mammary sentinel lymph nodes (T3/4 N1 M0).
Stage IV (metastatic cancer)	Regardless of the size of the tumour and the degree of nodal invasion, the presence of distant metastases classifies the cancer as stage IV (all T all N M1). Fixed axillary nodes, attachment of the tumour to the chest wall, supracalvicular nodes, skin metastases distant from the tumour, metastases in the other breast, various distant metastases.

Annex III

Table XXXII: pTNM classification of breast cancers and clinical stages (AJCC,8• 2017 edition).

Categories		Criteria
T	**TIS**	carcinoma in situ (pre-invasive) or nipple disease paget du with no detectable tumour.
	T0	no primary tumour.
	T1 (Tumour < 20 mm)	T1mi: microinvasive lesion < 1mm.
		T1a: 1mm < Tumour < 5mm.
		T1b:5mm < Tumour < 10mm.
		Tic:10mm < Tumour < 20mm.
	T2	20mm < T < 50mm.
	T3	Tumour > 50mm.
	T4 Tumour of any size extending to the chest wall (other than the pectoral muscle) or to the skin	T4a: extension to the chest wall. T4b: infiltrating skin ulceration (including peau d'orange) or skin nodules. T4c: extension to the skin and wall. T4d: infiammatone carcinoma.
N	**pN0**	No regional lymph node metastases detected on standard histology.
	pN1	pNimi: Micrometastasis (between 0.2 mm and/or more than 200 cells < 2.0mm).
		pN1a: Involvement of 1 to 3 axillary lymph nodes at least (including one metastasis > 2mm)
		pNib: Involvement of the internal mammary chain.
		pNic: pNia and pNib.
	pN2	pN2a: Involvement of 4 to 9 axillary lymph nodes at least (including one metastasis > 2mm)
		pN2b: Involvement of the internal mammary chain with a
		no axillary involvement
	pN3	pN3a: Involvement of at least 10 axillary lymph nodes
		pN3b:pN1a or pNa2 in the presence of clinical involvement of the internal chain / or pN2a and pN1b
		pN3c: Involvement of the homolateral supra-calvicular group
M	M0	No distant metastases.
	M1	existence of metastases (including skin nodules distant from the breast)

Annex IV

Table XXXIII: Clinical, histopathological and molecular characteristics of triple-negative breast cancer

Patient characteristics	-Young age at diagnosis: < 50 -High prevalence among African-Americans, Hispanics and sub-Saharans -First tumour in ***BRCA1*** mutation carriers	
Characteristics of the tumour	-Ductal histology: 80-93% ductal (CCI), 5% lobular, 4% metaplastic (aggressive, high grade, high mitotic activity and poor prognosis), 2.3% medullary (rare but good prognosis), 1.6% apocrine, 0.9% neuroendocrine, 0.5% cribiform and 0.5% mudneous -High histological grade: 77 to 90% grade III, 10% grade I - High mitotic index - Tumour size and the rate of positive lymph nodes are higher	
Molecular characteristics	Strong expression	EGFR (HERI) ; Basal cytokeratins (CK) 5,14 and 17 : Ki67 : c-Kit: Cyclin E; PI 6
	Weak expression	ER;PR;HER2;CyclinDl
Prognosis / Treatment	-Worst prognosis -Chinilo sensitivity prima ire No targeted therapy currently in use High risk of early relapse	

Annex V

Table XXXIV: Distribution of tumours by histological type according to age

Age					
		Frequency	Percentage	Valid percentage	Cumulative percentage
Valid	30	2	3,4	3,4	3,4
	32	1	1,7	1,7	5,1
	34	1	1,7	1,7	6,8
	35	1	1,7	1,7	8,5
	36	1	1,7	1,7	10,2
	37	3	5,1	5,1	15,3
	38	7	11,9	11,9	27,1
	39	6	10,2	10,2	37,3
	40	3	5,1	5,1	42,4
	41	4	6,8	6,8	49,2
	42	3	5,1	5,1	54,2
	43	2	3,4	3,4	57,6
	44	2	3,4	3,4	61,0
	45	5	8,5	8,5	69,5
	46	1	1,7	1,7	71,2
	47	2	3,4	3,4	74,6
	48	2	3,4	3,4	78,0
	49	4	6,8	6,8	84,7
	50	9	15,3	15,3	100,0
	Total	59	100,0	100,0	

Annex VI

Table XXXV :Table of clinicopathological parameters of patients studied with triple-negative breast cancer[2017 - 2022]

Patient number	Code	Age (years)	Sex e	Tumor a seat 1	Histological appearance	Tumour size	Grade of SBR	Clinical stage T	N	M	Type of surgery	lymph node invasion
1	H126	42	F	Left	CCI	2.5 X 1 X 2 cm	III	2	the	x	Mastectomy	EG +
2	H279	50	F	Left	CCL	5x3 cm	III	2	the	x	Mastectomy	EG +
3	H547	41	F	Law	CCI	1 X 1 X 2.5 cm	II	1b	0	x	Mastectomy	EG +
4	H869	30	F	Law	CCI	2 cm	II	the	3c	x	Mastectomy	EG +
5	H1682	43	F	Left	CCL	7x3 cm	III	2	the	1	Mastectomy	EG +
6	H1813	47	F	Law	CCI	3.5 X 2 X 2.5	III	2	the	1	Mastectomy	EG +
7	H2105	37	F	Law	CCL	1 X 1 X 2.5 cm	II	the	the	1	Mastectomy	EG +
8	H2150	38	F	Left	CCI	1.5 X 2 X 2.5 cm	II	2	0	x	Mastectomy	EG-
9	H2262	38	F	Law	CCI	1.5 X 2.2 X 2 cm	II	2	0	x	Mastectomy	EG +
10	H2263	45	F	Law	CCI	3 X 2.5 X 2 cm	II	2	0	x	Mastectomy	EG +
11	H2630	50	F	Left	CCI	2.5 X 1 X 2 cm	III	2	the	x	Mastectomy	EG +
12	IMN EXT	48	H	Left	CCI	5x2 cm	II	1b	0	x	Mastectomy	EG +
13	H130	50	F	Left	CCI	2 X 2 X 0.7 cm	II	2	0	x	Mastectomy	EG +
14	H199	37	F	Law	CCI	1.8 X 1.2 X 0.5 cm	II	the	the	x	Mastectomy	EG +
15	H347	38	F	Law	CCI	3.5 X 2.5 X 2.5 cm	II	2	0	x	Mastectomy	EG-
16	H576	42	F	Law	CCL	3x2x5 cm	III	2	the	x	Mastectomy	EG +
17	H737	38	F	Law	CCI	4 X 3 X 0.6 cm	III	2	3a	x	Mastectomy	EG+

18	H1929	36	F	Left	CCI	1 X 1 X 2.5 cm	II	1b	0	1	Mastectomy	EG +
19	H825	43	F	Law	CCI	0.3 ж 0.7 cm	III	2	0	x	Mastectomy	EG +
20	H1118	42	H	Left	CCI	3 X 2.5 cm	II	2	the	x	Mastectomy	EG +
21	H1526	35	F	Left	CCL	3 X 2.5 X 6 cm	III	2	the	x	Mastectomy	EG +
22	H1661	44	F	Left	CCI	1 X 1.5 X 2 cm	II	the	3c	x	Mastectomy	EG +
23	H1929	50	F	Left	CCI	1.5 X 1.5 X 1.5 cm	III	2	3a	x	Mastectomy	EG +
24	H2440	48	F	Left	CCI	3 X 2.5 X 3 cm	III	2	3a	x	Mastectomy	EG +
25	H2400	37	F	Law	CCI	3.5 X 3 X 3 cm	III	2	0	x	Mastectomy	EG +
26	H 2573	50	F	Law	CCI	2.5 X 2 X 0.9 cm	II	1	3c	x	Mastectomy	EG +
27	H 2792	44	F	Left	CCI	7x5x4 cm	III	1b	0	x	Mastectomy	EG +
28	H 2808	45	F	Law	CCI	4x2 cm	III	2	0	x	Mastectomy	EG +
29	H2884	40	F	Left	CCI	3x2 cm	III	2	1	x	Mastectomy	EG +
30	H3103	39	F	Left	CCI	7 cm	III	3	3a	x	Mastectomy	EG +
31	H2992	49	H	Law	CCI	4x3 cm	II	2	0	x	Tumorectomy	EG +
32	R43	30	F	Law	CCI	2.5 X 0.5 X 1cm	II	1b	1	x	Mastectomy	EG+
33	H586	39	F	Law	CCI / CCL	3.5 X 2 X 8 cm	II	2	the	x	Mastectomy	EG +
34	H264	47	H	Law	CCI	1.5 X 2 X 3.5 cm	III	3	the	x	Mastectomy	EG +
35	H2494	39	F	Left	CCI	2 X 2 X 1.5 cm	II	2	the	x	Mastectomy	EG +
36	H2695	40	F	Law	CCI	3 X 1.5 X 1.5 cm	II	1	the	x	Mastectomy	EG +
37	R02	50	F	Left	CCI	2.5 X 2.5 X 1 cm	II	2	0	x	Mastectomy	EG +
38	H140	41	F	Left	CCI	0.5 X 1 X 4 cm	II	0	2	1	Mastectomy	EG +
39	H158	50	F	Law	CCI	3.5 X 0.5 X 2.5 cm	II	2	0	x	Mastectomy	EG +
40	H167	41	F	Left	CCI	5x4x3 cm	III	2	1	x	Mastectomy	EG +

41	H172	38	F		Law	CCI	4x4x2 cm	II	2	th e	x	Mastectomy	EG +
42	H333	45	F		Law	CCI / CCL	3 cm	II	2	th e	x	Mastectomy	EG +
43	H521	45	F		Left	CCI	8x7 cm	II	3	2a	x	Mastectomy	EG +
44	H586	39	F		Law	CCI	3.5 X 2 cm	II	2	th e	x	Mastectomy	EG +
45	H1313	39	F		Law	CCI	2.5 X 2.5 X 1.5 cm	II	2	0	x	Mastectomy	EG +
46	H1795	38	F		Left	CCI	4.5 cm	II	2	0	x	Mastectomy	EG +
47	H2042	40	F		Law	CCI	5cm	II	2	0	x	Mastectomy	EG +
48	H2189	41	F		Left	CCI	2.5 cm	II	1c	0	x	Mastectomy	EG +
49	R05	39	F		Left	CCI	3.5 x 2.5 x 1.5 cm	II	2	th e	x	Mastectomy	EG +
50	R24	38	F		Left	CCI	3 X 3.5 X 4 cm	II	1c	1	x	Mastectomy	EG +
51	HIOO l	32	F		Left	CCI	3x3 cm	III	2	0	x	Mastectomy	EG +
52	H734	49	F		Left	CCI	3 X 2.5 cm	III	2	th e	x	Mastectomy	EG +
53	H2494	50	F		Law	CCI	3.5 X 3.5 X 3	II	2	th e	x	Mastectomy	EG +
54	H2459	49	F		Law	CCL	4x3 cm	II	4	2a	1	Mastectomy	EG +
55	B254	34	F		Left	CCI	3.5 X 2 cm	II	2	th e	x	Tumorectom y	EG-
56	B138	45	F		Left	CCI	4 x 3.5 cm	II	1c	0	x	Tumorectom y	EG-
57	B1051	46	F		Law	CCI	3.5 X 1 cm	II	2	th e	x	Tumorectom y	EG-
58	B91	49	F		Left	CCI	4.5 X 2.5 cm	II	1c	th e	x	Tumorectom y	EG-
59	B22	50	F		Law	CCI	3.5 cm	II	2	0	x	Tumorectom y	EG-

Annex VII

Table XXXVI: Clinicopathological characteristics of 480 patients with breast cancer in 2017-2022

Patients	480(100%)	
Gender	Male	8(1,66%)
	Female	472(98,33%)
Tumour site	Law	228(47,5%)
	Left	241(50,2%)
	Bilateral	11(2,29%)
Histological type	Lobular	62(12,91%)
	Ductal	399(83,12%)
	Other	19(3,95%)
Grade SBR	I	0(0%)
	II	282(58,75%)
	III	198(41,25%)
Tumour size	1	100(20,83%)
	2	260(54,16%)
	3	120(25%)
	4	0(0%)
Invasion of lymph nodes	NO	162(33,75%)
	N1	126(26,25%)
	N2	121(25,20%)
	N3	71(14,79%)
Remote metastasis	M0	216(45%)
	MI	16(3,33%)
	Mx	248 (51,66%)
Oestrogen receptor	positive	274(57,08%)
	negative	206(42,91%)
Progesterone receptor	Positive	264(55%)
	negative	216(45%)
HER2 status	Positive	182(37,91%)
	negative	298(62,08)
Molecular sub-type	Luminal A	136(28,33)
	Luminal B	103(21,45)
	HER2	182(37,91)
	Triple negative	59(12,29)

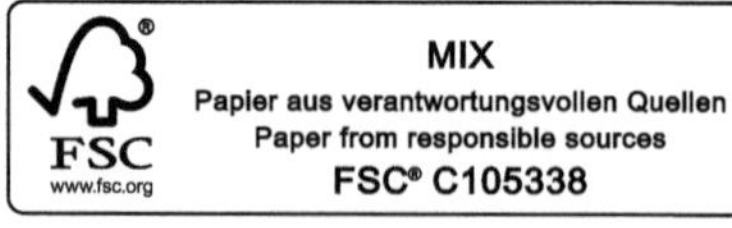

Printed by Books on Demand GmbH, Norderstedt / Germany